T0362485

Ablative Therapies in Neurosurgery

Editors

PETER NAKAJI
OLIVER BOZINOV

NEUROSURGERY
CLINICS OF NORTH AMERICA

www.neurosurgery.theclinics.com

Consulting Editors
RUSSELL R. LONSER
DANIEL K. RESNICK

April 2023 • Volume 34 • Number 2

ELSEVIER

1600 John F. Kennedy Boulevard • Suite 1800 • Philadelphia, Pennsylvania, 19103-2899

http://www.theclinics.com

NEUROSURGERY CLINICS OF NORTH AMERICA Volume 34, Number 2
April 2023 ISSN 1042-3680, ISBN-13: 978-0-443-18366-9

Editor: Stacy Eastman
Developmental Editor: Ann Gielou Posedio

Photocopying

Single photocopies of single articles may be made for personal use as allowed by national copyright laws. Permission of the Publisher and payment of a fee is required for all other photocopying, including multiple or systematic copying, copying for advertising or promotional purposes, resale, and all forms of document delivery. Special rates are available for educational institutions that wish to make photocopies for non-profit educational classroom use. For information on how to seek permission visit www.elsevier.com/permissions or call: (+44) 1865 843830 (UK)/(+1) 215 239 3804 (USA).

Derivative Works

Subscribers may reproduce tables of contents or prepare lists of articles including abstracts for internal circulation within their institutions. Permission of the Publisher is required for resale or distribution outside the institution. Permission of the Publisher is required for all other derivative works, including compilations and translations (please consult www.elsevier.com/permissions).

Electronic Storage or Usage

Permission of the Publisher is required to store or use electronically any material contained in this periodical, including any article or part of an article (please consult www.elsevier.com/permissions). Except as outlined above, no part of this publication may be reproduced, stored in a retrieval system or transmitted in any form or by any means, electronic, mechanical, photocopying, recording or otherwise, without prior written permission of the Publisher.

Notice

No responsibility is assumed by the Publisher for any injury and/or damage to persons or property as a matter of products liability, negligence or otherwise, or from any use or operation of any methods, products, instructions or ideas contained in the material herein. Because of rapid advances in the medical sciences, in particular, independent verification of diagnoses and drug dosages should be made.

Although all advertising material is expected to conform to ethical (medical) standards, inclusion in this publication does not constitute a guarantee or endorsement of the quality or value of such product or of the claims made of it by its manufacturer.

Neurosurgery Clinics of North America (ISSN 1042-3680) is published quarterly by Elsevier Inc., 360 Park Avenue South, New York, NY 10010-1710. Months of issue are January, April, July, and October. Business and Editorial Offices: 1600 John F. Kennedy Blvd., Suite 1800, Philadelphia, PA 19103-2899. Customer Service Office: 11830 Westline Industrial Drive, St. Louis, MO 63146. Periodicals postage paid at New York, NY, and additional mailing offices. Subscription prices are $451.00 per year (US individuals), $821.00 per year (US institutions), $484.00 per year (Canadian individuals), $1,019.00 per year (Canadian institutions), $562.00 per year (international individuals), $1,019.00 per year (international institutions), $100.00 per year (US students), $255.00 per year (international students), and $100.00 per year (Canadian students). International air speed delivery is included in all *Clinics* subscription prices. All prices are subject to change without notice. **POSTMASTER:** Send address changes to *Neurosurgery Clinics of North America*, Elsevier Periodicals Customer Service, 11830 Westline Industrial Drive, St. Louis, MO 63146. **Customer Service: 1-800-654-2452 (US and Canada). From outside the US and Canada, call: 1-314-453-7041. Fax: 1-314-453-5170. E-mail: JournalsCustomerService-usa@elsevier.com (for print support) and journalsonlinesupport-usa@elsevier.com (for online support).**

Reprints. For copies of 100 or more, of articles in this publication, please contact the Commercial Reprints Department, Elsevier Inc., 360 Park Avenue South, New York, NY 10010-1710. Tel. 212-633-3874; Fax: 212-633-3820; E-mail: reprints@elsevier.com.

Neurosurgery Clinics of North America is covered in *MEDLINE/PubMed (Index Medicus), EMBASE/Excerpta Medica, and Current Contents/Clinical Medicine (CC/CM).*

Contributors

CONSULTING EDITORS

RUSSELL R. LONSER, MD
Professor and Chair, Department of
Neurological Surgery, The Ohio State
University Wexner Medical Center, Columbus,
Ohio, USA

DANIEL K. RESNICK, MD, MS
Professor and Vice Chairman, Program
Director, Department of Neurosurgery,
University of Wisconsin-Madison School of
Medicine and Public Health, Madison,
Wisconsin, USA

EDITORS

PETER NAKAJI, MD
Chair, Department of Neurosurgery at Banner,
University Medical Center, Phoenix, Arizona,
USA

OLIVER BOZINOV, MD
Professor, Department of Neurosurgery,
Kantonsspital St. Gallen, St Gallen, Switzerland

AUTHORS

EVA C. ALDEN, PhD
Department of Psychiatry, Mayo Clinic,
Rochester, Minnesota, USA

MARIA ANASTASIADOU, PhD
Department of Neurological Surgery, Icahn
School of Medicine at Mount Sinai, New York,
New York, USA

ANILCHANDRA ATTALURI, PhD
Department of Mechanical Engineering,
The Pennsylvania State University,
Harrisburg, Middletown, Pennsylvania,
USA

JIRI BARTEK Jr, MD, PhD
Department of Clinical Neuroscience, Section
for Neurosurgery, Karolinska Institutet,
Department of Neurosurgery, Karolinska
University Hospital, Stockholm, Sweden;
Department of Neurosurgery, Rigshospitalet,
Copenhagen, Denmark

ALEXANDROS BOURAS, MD
Department of Neurological Surgery, University
of Pittsburgh, Brain Tumor Nanotechnology
Laboratory, UPMC Hillman Cancer Center,
Pittsburgh, Pennsylvania, USA

OLIVER BOZINOV, MD
Professor, Department of Neurosurgery,
Kantonsspital St. Gallen, St Gallen, Switzerland

DAVID B. BURKHOLDER, MD
Department of Neurology, Division of Epilepsy,
Mayo Clinic, Rochester, Minnesota, USA

ARPAN R. CHAKRABORTY, MD
Department of Neurological Surgery, University
Hospitals, Cleveland Medical Center, Case
Western Reserve University, School of
Medicine, Cleveland, Ohio, USA

CLARK C. CHEN, MD, PhD
Professor, Department of Neurological
Surgery, University of Minnesota, Minneapolis,
Minnesota, USA

DOMENICO CICALA, MD
Department of Pediatric Neurosurgery,
Santobono-Pausilipon Children's Hospital,
AORN, Napoli, Italy

GIUSEPPE CINALLI, MD, FACS
Department of Pediatric Neurosurgery,
Santobono-Pausilipon Children's Hospital,
AORN, Napoli, Italy

SHABBAR F. DANISH, MD, FAANS
Professor and Chairman, Department of Neurosurgery, Hackensack Meridian School of Medicine, Hackensack Meridian Health, Jersey Shore University Hospital, Jersey Shore University Medical Center, Neptune, New Jersey, USA

W. JEFFREY ELIAS, MD
Department of Neurosurgery, University of Virginia, School of Medicine, Charlottesville, Virginia, USA

CHRISTINA MALLING ENGELMANN, MSC
Clinical Neuropsychologist, Center for Neurorehabilitation, Lions Kollegiet, Copenhagen, Denmark

MICHAEL FAGERLUND, MD, PhD
Department of Neuroradiology, Karolinska University Hospital, Stockholm, Sweden

ALEXANDER FLETCHER-SANDERSJÖÖ, MD
Department of Clinical Neuroscience, Section for Neurosurgery, Karolinska Institutet, Department of Neurosurgery, Karolinska University Hospital, Stockholm, Sweden

SANGEET S. GREWAL, MD
Department of Neurosurgery Mayo Clinic, Jacksonville, Florida, USA

KLARA GUÐMUNDSDÓTTIR, MD
Department of Clinical Neuroscience, Section for Neurosurgery, Karolinska Institutet, Department of Neurosurgery, Karolinska University Hospital, Stockholm, Sweden

CONSTANTINOS G. HADJIPANAYIS, MD, PhD
Department of Neurological Surgery, Icahn School of Medicine at Mount Sinai, New York, New York, USA; Department of Neurological Surgery, University of Pittsburgh, Brain Tumor Nanotechnology Laboratory, UPMC Hillman Cancer Center, Pittsburgh, Pennsylvania, USA

MARWAN HARIZ, MD, PhD
Professor, Department of Clinical Neuroscience, University Hospital, Umea, Sweden

THOMAS HUNDSBERGER, MD
Departments of Neurology and Oncology, Kantonsspital St. Gallen, Medical School St. Gallen, St Gallen, Switzerland

AMNA HUSSEIN, MD
Research Fellow, Department of Neurosurgery at Banner, University Medical Center, Phoenix, Arizona, USA

ROBERT IVKOV, PhD
Department of Radiation Oncology and Molecular Radiation Sciences, Department of Oncology, Johns Hopkins School of Medicine, Departments of Mechanical Engineering, and Materials Science and Engineering, Johns Hopkins University, Whiting School of Engineering, Baltimore, Maryland, USA

ASGEIR S. JAKOLA, MD, PhD
Professor, Department of Clinical Neuroscience, Institute of Neuroscience and Physiology, Sahlgrenska Academy, Department of Neurosurgery, Sahlgrenska University Hospital, Gothenburg, Sweden

MARGRET JENSDOTTIR, MD
Department of Clinical Neuroscience, Section for Neurosurgery, Karolinska Institutet, Department of Neurosurgery, Karolinska University Hospital, Stockholm, Sweden

BO JESPERSEN, MD
Neurosurgeon, Head of Epilepsy Surgery, Department of Neurosurgery, Rigshospitalet, Copenhagen, Denmark

TIMOTHY J. KAUFMANN, MD, MS
Department of Radiology, Mayo Clinic, Rochester, Minnesota, USA

ANNIKA KITS, MD
Department of Neuroradiology, Karolinska University Hospital, Department of Clinical Neuroscience, Karolinska Institutet, Stockholm, Sweden

LAWRENCE KLEINBERG, MD
Department of Radiation Oncology and Molecular Radiation Sciences, Johns Hopkins University, Baltimore, Maryland, USA

MARIE KRÜGER, MD
Department of Neurosurgery, Kantonsspital St. Gallen, Medical School St. Gallen, St Gallen, Switzerland; Unit of Functional Neurosurgery, Institute of Neurology and Neurosurgery, London, United Kingdom; Department of Stereotactic and Functional Neurosurgery, University Medical Center Freiburg, Freiburg, Germany

DARA L. KRAITCHMAN, VMD, PhD, MS
Russell H. Morgan Department of Radiology and Radiological Science, Johns Hopkins University, Baltimore, Maryland, USA

VANCE T. LEHMAN, MD
Department of Radiology, Mayo Clinic, Rochester, Minnesota, USA

TOMAS MAJING, MD
Department of Perioperative Medicine and Intensive Care, Karolinska University Hospital, Stockholm, Sweden

ERIK H. MIDDLEBROOKS, MD
Department of Radiology, Mayo Clinic, Jacksonville, Florida, USA

JONATHAN P. MILLER, MD
Department of Neurological Surgery, University Hospitals, Cleveland Medical Center, Case Western Reserve University, School of Medicine, Cleveland, Ohio, USA

KAI J. MILLER, MD, PhD
Department of Neurosurgery Mayo Clinic, Rochester, Minnesota, USA

GIUSEPPE MIRONE, MD
Department of Pediatric Neurosurgery, Santobono-Pausilipon Children's Hospital, AORN, Napoli, Italy

SIGNE DELIN MOLDRUP, MSC
Clinical Neuropsychologist, Department of Neurosurgery, Rigshospitalet, Copenhagen East, Denmark

SHAYAN MOOSA, MD
Department of Neurosurgery, University of Virginia, School of Medicine, Charlottesville, Virginia, USA

PETER NAKAJI, MD
Chair, Department of Neurosurgery at Banner, University Medical Center, Phoenix, Arizona, USA

MARIAN CHRISTOPH NEIDERT, MD
Department of Neurosurgery, Kantonsspital St. Gallen, Medical School St. Gallen, St Gallen, Switzerland

SILAS HAAHR NIELSEN, MD
Pre-Residency Research and Clinical Fellow, Department of Neurosurgery, Rigshospitalet, Copenhagen East, Denmark

KRISTIN NOSOVA, MD, MBA
Resident, Department of Neurosurgery at Banner, University Medical Center, Phoenix, Arizona, USA

JONATHON J. PARKER, MD, PhD
Department of Neurosurgery Mayo Clinic, Scottsdale, Arizona, USA

NITESH V. PATEL, MD
Department of Neurosurgery, Hackensack Meridian School of Medicine, Hackensack Meridian Health, Jersey Shore University Hospital, Jersey Shore University Medical Center, Neptune, New Jersey, USA

PURVEE D. PATEL, MD
Department of Neurosurgery, Hackensack Meridian School of Medicine, Hackensack Meridian Health, Jersey Shore University Hospital, Jersey Shore University Medical Center, Neptune, New Jersey, USA

JONATHAN POMERANIEC, MD, MBA
Department of Neurosurgery, University of Virginia, School of Medicine, Charlottesville, Virginia, USA

ESTEBAN QUICENO, MD
Research Fellow, Department of Neurosurgery at Banner, University Medical Center, Phoenix, Arizona, USA

RUNE RASMUSSEN, MD, PhD
Neurosurgeon, Head of Stereotactic Team, Department of Neurosurgery, Rigshospitalet, Copenhagen East, Denmark

DANIEL RIVERA, BS
Department of Neurological Surgery, Icahn
School of Medicine at Mount Sinai, New York,
New York, USA; Department of Neurological
Surgery, University of Pittsburgh, Brain Tumor
Nanotechnology Laboratory, UPMC Hillman
Cancer Center, Pittsburgh, Pennsylvania,
USA

ULRIKA SANDVIK, MD, PhD
Department of Clinical Neuroscience, Section
for Neurosurgery, Karolinska Institutet,
Department of Neurosurgery, Karolinska
University Hospital, Stockholm,
Sweden

ALEXANDER J. SCHUPPER, MD
Department of Neurological Surgery, Icahn
School of Medicine at Mount Sinai, New York,
New York, USA

JANE SKJØTH-RASMUSSEN, MD, PhD
Neurosurgeon, Head of Brain Tumor Team,
Department of Neurosurgery, Rigshospitalet,
Copenhagen East, Denmark

KERRIN SUNSHINE, MD
Department of Neurological Surgery, University
Hospitals, Cleveland Medical Center, Case
Western Reserve University, School of
Medicine, Cleveland, Ohio, USA

JENNIFER A. SWEET, MD
Department of Neurological Surgery, University
Hospitals, Cleveland Medical Center, Case
Western Reserve University, School of
Medicine, Cleveland, Ohio, USA

SARA TABARI, MD
Department of Clinical Neuroscience, Section
for Neurosurgery, Karolinska Institutet,
Department of Neurosurgery, Karolinska
University Hospital, Stockholm, Sweden

ALEXIS PAUL ROMAIN TERRAPON, MD
Department of Neurosurgery, Kantonsspital St.
Gallen, Medical School St. Gallen, St Gallen,
Switzerland

JAMIE J. VAN GOMPEL, MD, FAANS
Department of Neurosurgery, Mayo Clinic,
Rochester, Minnesota, USA

Contents

 Video content accompanies this article at http://www.neurosurgery.theclinics.com.

> Real-time, MRI-guided laser interstitial thermal therapy (MRgLITT) is emerging as a minimally invasive technique for epilepsy surgery and for deep-seated tumors in the pediatric population. However, MRgLITT for posterior fossa lesions poses a unique challenge that is especially evident in this age range and remains understudied. In

this study, we report our experience and analyze the current literature on MRgLITT for the treatment of posterior fossa in children.

MR-guided laser interstitial thermal therapy (LITT) is feasible and safe in the awake patient. Awake LITT may be performed with analgesics for head fixation in a head-ring, no sedation during laser ablation, and with continuous neurological testing in patients with brain tumors and epilepsy. In the LITT treatment of lesions near eloquent areas and subcortical fiber tracts, neurological function can potentially be preserved by monitoring the patient during laser ablation.

Laser interstitial thermal therapy is an important new technique with a diverse use in epilepsy. This article gives an up-to-date evaluation of the current use of the technique within epilepsy, as well as provides some guidance to novice users appropriate clinical cases for its use.

A retrospective review of the first 30 patients treated with stereotactic laser ablation (SLA) at our institution since the introduction of the technique. We aimed to analyze initial results and learning curve. Indications were de novo gliomas (23%), recurrent gliomas (57%) and epileptogenic foci (20%). There was a trend towards improvement of lesion coverage and accuracy of catheter placement over time. Four patients (13.3%) experienced a new neurological deficit, where 3 patients had transient and 1 patient permanent deficits, respectively. Our results show a learning curve on precision measures over the first 30 cases.

Magnetic hyperthermia therapy (MHT) is a highly localized form of hyperthermia therapy (HT) that has been effective in treating various forms of cancer. Many clinical and preclinical studies have applied MHT to treat aggressive forms of brain cancer and assessed its role as a potential adjuvant to current therapies. Initial results show that MHT has a strong antitumor effect in animal studies and a positive association with overall survival in human glioma patients. Although MHT is a promising therapy with the potential to be incorporated into the future treatment of brain cancer, significant advancement of current MHT technology is required.

Current Applications of Ablative Therapies for Trigeminal Neuralgia 285

Arpan R. Chakraborty, Kerrin Sunshine, Jonathan P. Miller, and Jennifer A. Sweet

Trigeminal neuralgia (TN) is a painful condition affecting the trigeminal nerve. The etiology of TN has not been definitively established but is thought to involve neurovascular compression of the trigeminal nerve at the trigeminal root entry zone. Patients who do not respond to medical management may benefit from focal injury to the trigeminal nerve. Many lesions have been described, targeting fibers of the trigeminal nerve at various anatomical locations across its course. This article reviews the relevant anatomy and lesioning procedures for the treatment of trigeminal neuralgia.

Pros and Cons of Ablation for Functional Neurosurgery in the Neurostimulation Age 291

Marwan Hariz

Should one recommend stereotactic ablation for Parkinson disease, tremor, dystonia, and obsessive compulsive disorder, in this era of DBS? The answer depends on several variables such as the symptoms to treat, the patient's preferences and expectations, the surgeons' competence and preference, the availability of financial means (by government health care, by private insurance), the geographical issues, and not least the current and dominating fashion at that particular time. Both ablation and stimulation can be either used alone or even combined (provided expertise in both of them) to treat various symptoms of movement and mind disorders.

High-Frequency Ultrasound Ablation in Neurosurgery 301

Jonathan Pomeraniec, W. Jeffrey Elias, and Shayan Moosa

Modern transcranial magnetic resonance-guided focused ultrasound is an incisionless, ablative treatment modality for a growing number of neurologic disorders. This procedure selectively destroys a targeted volume of cerebral tissue and relies on real-time MR thermography to monitor tissue temperatures. By focusing on a submillimeter target through a hemispheric phased array of transducers, ultrasound waves pass through the skull and avoid overheating and brain damage. High-intensity focused ultrasound techniques are increasingly used to create safe and effective stereotactic ablations for medication-refractory movement and other neurologic and psychiatric disorders.

NEUROSURGERY CLINICS OF NORTH AMERICA

SERIES OF RELATED INTEREST

Neurologic Clinics
https://www.neurologic.theclinics.com/
Neuroimaging Clinics
https://www.neuroimaging.theclinics.com/

THE CLINICS ARE AVAILABLE ONLINE!
Access your subscription at:
www.theclinics.com

Preface
Ablation Therapies in Neurosurgery

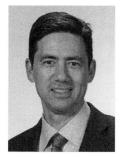   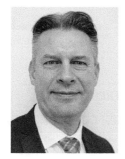

Peter Nakaji, MD   Oliver Bozinov, MD
Editors

The concept of localization of function in neurology and neurosurgery is owed to a series of early thinkers, including Gall, whose discredited theory of phrenology posited that bumps on the head had specific correlations and relations to brain functions. By the time of Broca, the concept that there was regionality in the brain was growing. Edwin Boldrey's description of the sensorimotor homunculus in his 1936 McGill master's degree thesis (supervised by Wilder Penfield) firmly entrenched the idea of specific localization in the neurosurgical psyche.[1] With that idea comes the parallel concept that certain pathologic conditions can be addressed by destroying certain structures that give rise to them, to wit, by ablation. By successive iteration defining targets and developing technology, ablation therapies are now a vital part of the neurosurgical toolkit that can achieve cellular inactivation of tumors, structures, or pathways to achieve clinical goals.

The articles in this issue provide a broad overview, in places more sweepingly and in others more in-depth, of the current state of application of ablation therapies. The journey begins with a concise history of how we came to current ablation therapies. How we have evolved from the earliest stages of ablation therapies, what we have retired or abandoned, and how we developed our current technologies inform where we

still may go. Among classic technologies, a review of the current application of ablation for trigeminal neuralgia anchors the list. Laser interstitial thermal therapy (LITT) has become the most widespread of the newer technologies and claims the lion's share of attention now. By delivering heat energy precisely in a way that can be monitored, LITT allows us to achieve targeted and tailored cell death in a way that has reinvigorated ablation in neurosurgery. Applications such as brain metastases, radionecrosis, and glioma are all detailed here by our colleagues, who are respected authorities in the field.

This issue also covers topics of application in specialized populations, such as LITT in the pediatric population and the performance of awake LITT. These are topics that are important because they open the technology to subgroups where the minimally invasive nature of the technique is particularly attractive.

Other topics include technologies that many have heard of but may not yet have a deep familiarity with, including MRI-guided high-frequency ultrasound ablation and magnetic hyperthermia.

Ablation therapies are here to stay for the duration. They satisfy multiple previously unmet needs, including the ability to treat effectively deep targets with a minimally invasive technique, the use

Neurosurg Clin N Am 34 (2023) xi–xii
https://doi.org/10.1016/j.nec.2023.01.002
1042-3680/23/© 2023 Published by Elsevier Inc.

of nonionizing radiation, and generally a favorable patient experience. Advances in the underlying technologies for delivering the ablation have been paced by the necessary techniques for real-time monitoring of the process. Nonetheless, opportunities for the field still remain. Further developments to improve the ability to treat larger lesions, to treat irregularly shaped lesions, and to interrupt networks in a rational range will be a welcomed part of technologies still to come. This issue represents a view into both the best practices of today and the promises of tomorrow.

Peter Nakaji, MD
Department of Neurosurgery at Banner
University Medical Center
755 East McDowell Road, 2nd Floor
Phoenix, AZ 85006, USA

Oliver Bozinov, MD
Department of Neurosurgery at
Kantonsspital St. Gallen
Klinik für Neurochirurgie
St. Gallen CH-9000
Switzerland

E-mail addresses:
peter.nakaji@bannerhealth.com (P. Nakaji)
oliver.bozinov@kssg.ch (O. Bozinov)

REFERENCE

1. Gandhoke GS, Belykh E, Zhao X, et al. Edwin Boldrey and Wilder Penfield's Homunculus: A Life Given by Mrs. Cantlie (In and Out of Realism). World Neurosurgery 2019;132:377–88.

History of Ablation Therapies in Neurosurgery

Kristin Nosova, MD, MBA[a], Esteban Quiceno, MD[a], Amna Hussein, MD[a], Oliver Bozinov, MD[b], Peter Nakaji, MD[a],*

KEYWORDS

- LITT • Neuroablation • Focused ultrasound thermal ablation • Laser interstitial thermal therapy

KEY POINTS

- Neuroablation techniques have undergone a recent renaissance, with laser interstitial thermal therapy (LITT) and high-intensity focused ultrasound (HIFU) emerging as promising techniques.
- Development of laser penetration technologies and MR thermography contributed to wide adoption of these technologies.
- LITT and HIFU have applications and shown clinical efficacy in the treatment of glioblastoma, metastasis, radiation necrosis, epilepsy, essential tremor, and chronic pain.
- Given the technological advances of the past 15 years, the coming years hold much promise for these techniques.

Neuroablation techniques have undergone a recent renaissance that has placed ablation firmly back into the modern neurosurgical armamentarium. The techniques that have been developed for tissue ablation over the past several decades aim for the selective destruction of cerebral tissue and/or interruption of maladaptive cerebral networks.[1]

Multiple physical principles have been used for brain tissue ablation: electromagnetic waves, chemical agents, ionizing radiation, induction of heat or cryogenics; high-intensity focused ultrasound, and radiofrequency.[1,2]

More recent and promising techniques include laser interstitial thermal therapy (LITT) (**Fig. 1**) and high-intensity focused ultrasound thermal ablation (HIFU).[1,2] We will focus primarily on these techniques in this brief historical review.

EARLY-STAGE LIMITATION OF LASER INTERSTITIAL THERMAL THERAPY

The concept of LITT for tumors has existed since the late 1970s. This treatment relies on the principle of delivering high-intensity electromagnetic radiation at varying wavelengths, power densities, durations, and methods of exposure.[3] This technique has been of limited use in intracranial disease due to underdeveloped imaging technology, which affected targeting and the ability to monitor thermal effects.

During the 1970s, three types of laser therapies were described: carbon dioxide laser (wavelength 10600 nm in the far infrared), the Nd:YAG (neodymium-doped yttrium aluminum garnet) laser (wavelength 1060 nm in the near-infrared), and the Argon ion laser with two main lines (at 488 and 514 nm) in the blue and green regions of the visible spectrum. In animal models, the Nd:YAG laser could be centered on any spot accessible to a single fiber within the surface of an organ. The extent and severity of laser damage depended on the energy dissipated and was reasonably predictable for each tissue. Laser treatments were observed to replace functioning tissue (normal or neoplastic) with fibrous tissue without affecting the mechanical integrity of the organ.[4]

[a] Department of Neurosurgery at Banner, University Medical Center, 755 East McDowell Road 2nd Floor, Phoenix, AZ 85006, USA; [b] Department of Neurosurgery, Kantonsspital St. Gallen, St Gallen CH-9000, Switzerland
* Corresponding author.
E-mail address: peter.nakaji@bannerhealth.com

Neurosurg Clin N Am 34 (2023) 193–198
https://doi.org/10.1016/j.nec.2022.12.002
1042-3680/23/© 2022 Elsevier Inc. All rights reserved.

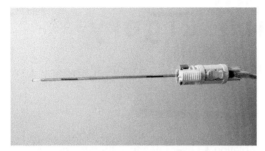

Fig. 1. One of the commercially available laser interstitial ablation probes.

EARLY USE OF LASER INTERSTITIAL THERMAL THERAPY IN HUMANS

Sugiyama and colleagues[5] used adult cats to examine the histological changes following laser hyperthermia. Under general anesthesia, a burr hole was made over the frontal hemisphere and a 5 mm contact probe with a frosted tip was inserted stereotactically into the basal ganglia. The thermal therapy was maintained between 42.5 and 43.5°C over 30 min of irradiation at 2 to 3 W. The center of the resultant lesion consisted of coagulation necrosis surrounded by a thin edematous zone contained within the heated area.

In the same article, the authors described the first reported use of LITT in treating brain tumors in humans. Five patients, three with gliomas and two with metastatic lesions, were treated with laser hyperthermia for 30 to 40 min at 2 to 3 W to maintain a temperature of 42.5°C to 43.5°C. No surgical complications were reported after the procedures. Subsequent studies reported good tumor control and favorable complication profile, although a lack of sophisticated laser probes with built-in cooling systems and unavailability of intraoperative thermal monitoring prevented the widespread adoption of this technique.

Early application of LITT was restricted to smaller lesions, but advances in optical fiber technology and development of a cooling mechanism allowed it to be extended to larger ones. This problem was overcome with the development of a cooling mechanism that takes the form of a sheath-like device that cools the optical fiber with a constant stream of fluid or cooled gas. The cooling mechanism removes heat from the probe tissue interface and minimizes vaporization or carbonization, allowing for larger treated volumes.[2]

After the initial experiments involving humans were published in the early 1990s, more studies reporting the outcome of laser ablation of high-grade gliomas were published. Reimer and colleagues[6] reported the outcomes of four patients with high-grade gliomas treated with LITT, with good local tumor control at 6-month follow-up.

Leonardi and colleagues[7] reported the outcomes of 24 patients (7 low-grade gliomas, 11 anaplastic gliomas, and 6 glioblastomas), most with recurrences before LITT. Mean survival after treatment was 34 months, 30 months, and 9 months, respectively; mean times to progression after LITT were 16 months, 10 months, and 4 months, respectively. This series reported one infection and two instances of new neurological deficit.

The development of lasers of different wavelengths improved treating times and made this technology available for fragile patients who would not tolerate a conventional open procedure. Importantly, the use of a 980-nm laser shortened the surgical time; a 2.5 cm metastatic lesion would require a 16-min ablation by radiofrequency, 73 min with a 1064 nm Nd:YAG laser, but only 6 min with a 980-nm laser.[8]

MR-GUIDED LASER INTERSTITIAL THERMAL THERAPY FOR BRAIN NEOPLASMS

Jethwa and colleagues[8] reported the outcomes of 20 patients with different types of brain tumors (ependymoma, meningioma, glioblastoma, hemangioblastoma, metastasis, and chordoma) treated with LITT in different locations, including the posterior fossa. In this case series, an MRI with real-time temperature map and estimates of tissue coagulation during the ablation process was used to avoid thermal injury of healthy brain tissue. Patients were considered for treatment if they had recurrence after previous surgical resection, tumors in inaccessible areas, and if they were considered high-risk surgical candidates. The average volume of the treated tumors was 7 ± 9 cm^3 (0.37 to 68.9 cm^3). The average power and procedure time during each ablation were 11 ± 1.4 W and 13.9 ± 10.7 min (range 1.38 to 35.9 min). Four patients presented perioperative complications. There was one arterial injury requiring operative repair, one case of severe edema requiring hemicraniectomy, and two complications due to poor placement of the laser probe.

Mohammadi and colleagues[9] reported 34 patients with high-grade gliomas who underwent LITT and showed that a higher percentage of contrast-enhancing tumor ablation was associated with increased survival. The authors proposed that the coverage of tumor volume by the hyperthermic field could be considered analogous to the "extent of resection" in the treatment of high-grade gliomas.

Mohammadi and colleagues[10] compared the outcomes of 24 patients with high-grade gliomas treated with LITT followed with chemo/radiotherapy and 24 patients treated with biopsy followed by chemo/radiotherapy. The median estimate of overall survival and progression-free survival in the LITT cohort was 14.4 and 4.3 months, respectively, compared with 15.8 and 5.9 months for the biopsy-only cohort. These findings suggest that the LITT therapy is an excellent option for patients with high-grade gliomas who are not considered good surgical candidates for gross total resection due to their clinical condition.

LASER INTERSTITIAL THERMAL THERAPY TO TREAT RADIATION NECROSIS

Stereotactic radiosurgery (SRS) alone or as adjuvant therapy has gained support in the management of intracranial primary and metastatic lesions over whole-brain radiation, with good safety and efficacy.[11] Radiation necrosis (RN), however, is a delayed adverse consequence of radiation therapy and can present as either an enhancing lesion on an MRI in an asymptomatic patients or as a worsening of preexisting symptoms, cognitive decline, headache, drowsiness, or memory loss.[12] Although the precise mechanisms underlying RN remain under investigation, there is evidence to suggest that RN is caused by vascular damage and subsequent immune activation resulting in edema, ischemia, and necrosis, with an incidence rate of up to 24% of treated lesions.[13] Traditionally, RN treatment centered around controlling vasogenic edema with corticosteroids and other therapies such as hyperbaric oxygen and anticoagulation, with mixed success rates. More recently, the anti-vascular endothelial growth factor antibody bevacizumab has been used to treat RN with response rates of 90%; however, this drug is costly, requires long-term use, and is associated with potentially severe side effects.[14]

Rahmathulla and colleagues[12] published the first report of a patient with medically refractory RN in a region not amenable to surgical decompression who was treated with LITT. They hypothesized that LITT would be able to replace the endothelial proliferating cells and zone of disorganized angiogenesis through thermal damage. The procedure was tolerated well and the patient was discharged 48 h postoperatively, with near complete resolution of the edema and associated mass effect at 7-week follow-up. This study

opened the door to new possibilities for the use of LITT.

Re-radiation of RN is associated with worsening disease and management of edema does not address any potential underlying tumor recurrence. LITT is an attractive treatment modality in this patient population as it has been shown to be effective for RN and tumor recurrence, and the method allows for a simultaneous stereotactic biopsy during probe placement. LITT has been shown to relieve RN symptoms, reduce progression, and improve survival in patients with RN and brain metastases. Rao and colleagues[15] reported local control rate of 75% at 24 weeks, and median progression-free survival of 37 weeks. Several studies reported similar effectiveness for LITT versus craniotomy for recurrent lesions (RN and/or tumor). Additionally, LITT has consistently been associated with shorter length of stay and less perioperative pain.

LASER INTERSTITIAL THERMAL THERAPY FOR EPILEPSY

Victor Horsley described a successful localization and resection of an epileptogenic focus resulting in seizure freedom in a patient over 100 years ago.[13] Since then, multiple neurosurgical techniques have been developed to treat refractory epilepsy. Anterior temporal lobectomy (ATL) and selective amygdalohippocampectomy (SAH) are the two most common epilepsy procedures both resulting in >70% seizure freedom, although SAH has been associated with superior neurocognitive outcomes.[16] The observation that less invasive approaches and preservation of more normal anatomy might result in fewer postoperative deficits led clinicians to search for minimally invasive techniques.[17] As more predictable laser penetration technologies and MR thermography were developed, MRI-guided laser ablation became a promising minimal-invasive alternative to traditional ATL and SAH, targeting the same anatomy with laser probes instead of open techniques. Studies in patients with mesial temporal sclerosis comparing LITT with an open resection reported lower seizure freedom between 50% and 67% (Engel I) at 6 and 12 months with superior complications profile, lower postoperative pain, shorter hospital stay, and faster recovery.[16]

LASER INTERSTITIAL THERMAL THERAPY FOR HYPOTHALAMIC HAMARTOMA

Hypothalamic hamartomas (HH) are rare congenital, nonneoplastic, neuroglial lesions of the ventral hypothalamus localized to the tuber cinereum on the floor of the third ventricle. These lesions present with gelastic seizures due to proximity to mammillary bodies and/or precocious puberty caused by premature secretion of gonadotropin-releasing hormone. The disease has a disabling course, marked by intractable seizures, cognitive decline, and psychiatric symptoms.

Despite advances in HH surgery over the years, traditional approaches have continued to be plagued with mixed results. The anterior interhemispheric transcallosal approach results in Engel I and Engel II outcomes in 51% and 24% of patients, respectively, but is also associated with significant complication rates such as memory deficits (30% to 50%) and hypothalamic obesity (45%). Similarly, the endoscopic approach is associated with Engel I and Engel II outcomes in 46% and 24% of patients, respectively, and has complication rates of 8% for memory dysfunction and 30% for stroke.[18] Radiosurgery is associated with a complete seizure freedom rate of less than 40%.[19]

With the advent of MR thermography that allows for visualization of temperature changes within a large scanned field, LITT was promoted as a minimally invasive alternative for the treatment of HH.[20] The efficacy is derived from both destruction and disconnection of epileptogenic tissue, with the goal of preventing propagation of seizures into either mammillary bodies or the hypothalamus. The procedure can be performed using several workflow paradigms with frame-based or frameless stereotaxy for the placement of laser fiber within the cooling cannula into the target via an avascular trajectory, followed by MR-guided thermal ablation.

On the basis of a recent meta-analysis by Barot and colleagues,[21] 67% of patients who underwent LITT for HH experience seizure freedom (Engel I), with the overall complication rate of 19% after 10 months of follow-up.

HIGH-INTENSITY FOCUSED ULTRASOUND THERMAL ABLATION

The interest in sound waves dates back to Aristotle's theory of propagation via air particles. Ultrasonic waves are sound waves that propagate through matter with frequencies above the hearing range of human ears (>20,000 Hz). Medical use of ultrasound transducers started in the 1930s after it was applied to the management of rheumatoid arthritis. Currently, transcranial treatments are performed with a focused piezoelectric transducer that converges ultrasonic energy (1 to 3 MHz) onto a target tissue producing localized tissue destruction. The focal zone is defined as the area

where the ultrasound intensity is high enough to create a lesion that is ellipsoidal, approximately 8 to 15 mm in length, with a diameter of 1 to 2 mm. The exposure can be constant (thermal) or pulsed (acoustic cavitation). Ultrasound produces frictional heat by causing vibration of molecules in a determined tissue; a temperature of more than 56°C for 2 s or more produces coagulative necrosis.[22]

In 2001 the first integrated MR-guided Focused Ultrasound (MRgFUS) machine was designed. In 2006, Ram and colleagues[23] published the first report on MRgFUS, which included three patients with glioblastoma. Initially, the patients required craniectomy 7 to 10 days before the procedure to create a bony window for the ultrasound treatment. MRgFUS treatment resulted in immediate radiological changes and subsequent evidence of thermocoagulation.

Martin and colleagues[24] reported the use of MRgFUS in nine patients with chronic pain who underwent ablation of the posterior part of the thalamic central lateral nucleus using a completely noninvasive technique. Patients were fully awake and responsive during all stages of the intervention. Relief of pain after the intervention ranged from 20% to 100% with a mean of 68% and no surgical-related complications were recorded.

Since then, there have been multiple reports of the use of this technology for the treatment of intracerebral hemorrhage, Parkinson's disease, and essential tremors.[25–27]

Elias and colleagues[28] published a landmark article about the use of MRgFUS in functional pathologies, describing 76 patients with moderate to severe essential tremor who did not respond to at least two trials of medical therapy and were randomly assigned in a 3:1 ratio to undergo unilateral focused ultrasound thalamotomy or a sham procedure. A total of 56 patients underwent thalamotomy. The hand tremor scores improved significantly in the thalamotomy group and secondary outcomes such as disability and quality of life also improved after the procedure. Adverse events in the thalamotomy group included gait disturbance in 36% of patients and paresthesias or numbness in 38%, these adverse events persisted at 12 months in 9% and 14% of patients, respectively.

Currently, this technology is one of the many options to treat patients with glioblastoma and other malignant brain tumors through mediated hyperthermia, stimulation of the immune system to target tumor cells, and administration of sonosensitizers that produce reactive oxygen species (ROS) and contribute to tumor apoptosis in the presence of focus ultrasound. This technology

RESULTS BY YEAR

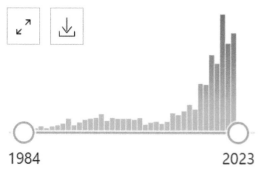

1984   2023

Fig. 2. Publications for the keywords "laser interstitial thermal therapy" on Pubmed.gov.

may play a critical role in the treatment of patients with malignant brain tumors.[11]

SUMMARY

LITT and HIFU are treatment options with great potential to treat glioblastoma, metastasis, epilepsy, essential tremor, and chronic pain. Results from recent studies show that LITT is a viable alternative to conventional surgical techniques in select patient populations. Although many of the bases for these treatments have existed since the 1930s, the most important advancement in these techniques has occurred in the last 15 years and, based on the large rise in publication volume (**Fig. 2**), the coming years hold much promise for these treatments.

CLINICS CARE POINTS

- Laser interstitial thermal therapy (LITT) therapy is an excellent option for patients with high-grade gliomas who are not considered good surgical candidates for gross total resection.

- There is evidence of clinical equipoise for LITT for radiation necrosis and recurrent metastatic disease, with shorter length of stay and less perioperative pain among patients with LITT.

- Mesial temporal sclerosis patients treated with LITT versus resection have lower seizure freedom between 50% and 67% (vs 60% to 80% for traditional anterior temporal lobectomy and selective amygdalohippocampectomy) but with quicker recovery and superior complications profiles.

DISCLOSURE

The authors have nothing to disclose.

REFERENCES

1. Franzini A, Moosa S, Servello D, et al. Ablative brain surgery: an overview. Int J Hyperthermia 2019;36(2): 64–80.
2. Missios S, Bekelis K, Barnett GH. Renaissance of laser interstitial thermal ablation. Neurosurg Focus 2015;38(3):E13.
3. Mirza FA, Mitha R, Shamim MS. Current Role of Laser Interstitial Thermal Therapy in the Treatment of Intracranial Tumors. Asian J Neurosurg 2020; 15(4):800–8.
4. Bown SG. Phototherapy in tumors. World J Surg 1983;7(6):700–9.
5. Sugiyama K, Sakai T, Fujishima I, et al. Stereotactic interstitial laser-hyperthermia using Nd-YAG laser. Stereotact Funct Neurosurg 1990;54-55:501–5.
6. Reimer P, Bremer C, Horch C, et al. MR-monitored LITT as a palliative concept in patients with high grade gliomas: preliminary clinical experience. J Magn Reson Imaging 1998;8(1):240–4.
7. Leonardi MA, Lumenta CB. Stereotactic guided laser-induced interstitial thermotherapy (SLITT) in gliomas with intraoperative morphologic monitoring in an open MR: clinical expierence. Minim Invasive Neurosurg 2002;45(4):201–7.
8. Jethwa PR, Barrese JC, Gowda A, et al. Magnetic resonance thermometry-guided laser-induced thermal therapy for intracranial neoplasms: initial experience. Neurosurgery 2012;71(1 Suppl Operative): 133–44, 144-144.
9. Mohammadi AM, Hawasli AH, Rodriguez A, et al. The role of laser interstitial thermal therapy in enhancing progression-free survival of difficult-to-access high-grade gliomas: a multicenter study. Cancer Med 2014;3(4):971–9.
10. Mohammadi AM, Sharma M, Beaumont TL, et al. Upfront magnetic resonance imaging-guided stereotactic laser-ablation in newly diagnosed glioblastoma: a multicenter review of survival outcomes compared with a matched cohort of biopsy-only patients. Neurosurgery 2019;85(6):762–72.
11. Hersh AM, Bhimreddy M, Weber-Levine C, et al. Applications of focused ultrasound for the treatment of glioblastoma: a new frontier. Cancers (Basel) 2022; 14(19):4920.
12. Bastos DCA, Weinberg J, Kumar VA, et al. Laser Interstitial Thermal Therapy in the treatment of brain metastases and radiation necrosis. Cancer Lett 2020;489:9–18.
13. Lee D, Riestenberg RA, Haskell-Mendoza A, et al. Brain Metastasis Recurrence Versus Radiation

Necrosis: Evaluation and Treatment. Neurosurg Clin N Am 2020;31(4):575–87.

14. Miyatake S, Nonoguchi N, Furuse M, et al. Pathophysiology, diagnosis, and treatment of radiation necrosis in the brain. Neurol Med Chir (Tokyo) 2015; 55(1):50–9.

15. Rahmathulla G, Recinos PF, Valerio JE, et al. Laser interstitial thermal therapy for focal cerebral radiation necrosis: a case report and literature review. Stereotact Funct Neurosurg 2012;90(3): 192–200.

16. Zemmar A, Nelson BJ, Neimat JS. Laser thermal therapy for epilepsy surgery: current standing and future perspectives. Int J Hyperthermia 2020;37(2): 77–83.

17. Hu WH, Zhang C, Zhang K, et al. Selective amygdalohippocampectomy versus anterior temporal lobectomy in the management of mesial temporal lobe epilepsy: a meta-analysis of comparative studies. J Neurosurg 2013;119(5):1089–97.

18. Ng YT, Rekate HL, Prenger EC, et al. Transcallosal resection of hypothalamic hamartoma for intractable epilepsy. Epilepsia 2006;47(7):1192–202.

19. Mithani K, Neudorfer C, Boutet A, et al. Surgical targeting of large hypothalamic hamartomas and seizure-freedom following MR-guided laser interstitial thermal therapy. Epilepsy Behav 2021;116: 107774.

20. Tzourio-Mazoyer N, Landeau B, Papathanassiou D, et al. Automated anatomical labeling of activations in SPM using a macroscopic anatomical parcellation of the MNI MRI single-subject brain. Neuroimage 2002;15(1):273–89.

21. Barot N, Batra K, Zhang J, et al. Surgical outcomes between temporal, extratemporal epilepsies and hypothalamic hamartoma: systematic review and meta-analysis of MRI-guided laser interstitial thermal therapy for drug-resistant epilepsy. J Neurol Neurosurg Psychiatry 2022;93(2):133–43.

22. Quadri SA, Waqas M, Khan I, et al. High-intensity focused ultrasound: past, present, and future in neurosurgery. Neurosurg Focus 2018;44(2):E16.

23. Ram Z, Cohen ZR, Harnof S, et al. Magnetic resonance imaging-guided, high-intensity focused ultrasound for brain tumor therapy. Neurosurgery 2006; 59(5):949–55 [discussion: 955-6].

24. Martin E, Jeanmonod D, Morel A, et al. High-intensity focused ultrasound for noninvasive functional neurosurgery. Ann Neurol 2009;66(6):858–61.

25. Elias WJ, Huss D, Voss T, et al. A pilot study of focused ultrasound thalamotomy for essential tremor. N Engl J Med 2013;369:640–8.

26. Harnof S, Zibly Z, Hananel A, et al. Potential of magnetic resonance-guided focused ultrasound for intracranial hemorrhage: an in vivo feasibility study. J Stroke Cerebrovasc Dis 2014;23:1585–91.

27. Magara A, Bühler R, Moser D, et al. First experience with MR-guided focused ultrasound in the treatment of Parkinson's disease. J Ther Ultrasound 2014;2:11.

28. Elias WJ, Lipsman N, Ondo WG, et al. A randomized trial of focused ultrasound thalamotomy for essential tremor. N Engl J Med 2016;375(8):730–9.

The Evolution of Laser-Induced Thermal Therapy for the Treatment of Gliomas

Purvee D. Patel, MD[a,b], Nitesh V. Patel, MD[a,b], Shabbar F. Danish, MD[a,b],*

KEYWORDS

- Laser-induced thermal therapy (LITT) • High-grade gliomas • Glioblastomas • Cytoreduction

KEY POINTS

- Although laser-induced thermal therapy (LITT) initially was used as a salvage treatment of recurrent gliomas that had exhausted standard treatment of care, it has evolved into a first-line treatment of specific newly diagnosed high-grade gliomas.
- LITT has comparable results to surgical debulking in allowing maximal cytoreduction, minimizing new neurologic deficits, prolonging malignant transformation, and improving overall and progression-free survival.

INTRODUCTION

As with most novel techniques, laser-induced thermal therapy (LITT) was initially met with some skepticism for its role in the treatment for intracranial pathologies. Over the last two decades, with the help of real-time monitoring, the use of LITT has expanded to a range of pathologies including intracranial metastases, gliomas, radiation necrosis, epilepsy, and so forth.[1] Initial use was typically limited—it was a salvage option for tumors, when the standard approach failed. However, as more neurosurgeons used LITT, its efficacy was obvious. With time, LITT has emerged as a favorable treatment, possibly even first line for certain pathologies. In glioma management, there has been an increasing favorability for LITT to even being considered comparable to current "standards of care" of both newly diagnosed and recurrent cases.

NATURAL DISEASE COURSE OF GLIOMAS

Gliomas can be characterized as low grade and high grade. Diffuse low-grade gliomas (DLGGs) typically have a peak onset at the age of about 35 to 40 years. They tend to have a slow growing, "silent" phase during which they could be found incidentally on imaging. This is followed by a symptomatic phase and then a progressive phase which is often precipitated by transformation to malignant, more high-grade gliomas.[2] The median survival in patients with low-grade astrocytomas is about 5 years and death usually results due to malignant transformation.[3]

High-grade or malignant gliomas are much more aggressive in their behavior and associated with a poorer prognosis. Of note, about 80% of high-grade, or malignant, gliomas are glioblastomas (GBMs) and represent the most common primary intracranial tumor in adults.[4] There are increasing molecular data that is being reported suggesting

ᵃ Department of Neurosurgery, Hackensack Meridian School of Medicine, Hackensack Meridian Health - Jersey Shore University Medical Center, Nutley, NJ 07110, USA; ᵇ Department of Neurosurgery, Hackensack Meridian School of Medicine, Hackensack Meridian Health, Jersey Shore University Hospital, Jersey Shore University Medical Center, 19 Davis Avenue, Hope Tower 4th Floor, Neptune, NJ 07753, USA
* Corresponding author. Department of Neurosurgery, Hackensack Meridian School of Medicine, Hackensack Meridian Health, Jersey Shore University Hospital, Jersey Shore University Medical Center, 19 Davis Avenue, Hope Tower 4th Floor, Neptune, NJ 07753.
E-mail address: shabbar.danish@hmhn.org

Neurosurg Clin N Am 34 (2023) 199–207
https://doi.org/10.1016/j.nec.2022.12.004
1042-3680/23/Published by Elsevier Inc.

subgroups may survive longer.[5,6] The peak onset for anaplastic astrocytoma is usually at age 40 to 50 years, whereas for GBMs, it is 60 to 70 years.[3] Primary GBMs tend to occur in older patients (mean age 55), whereas for secondary GBM, it is in younger adults (<45). The medial survival, despite aggressive treatment, is approximately 3 years for anaplastic astrocytomas and 1 year for GBMs.[3]

TREATMENT OF GLIOMAS AND THE CONCEPT OF CYTOREDUCTION

The standard of care for gliomas, especially high-grade gliomas such as GBMs, is surgical resection with adjuvant chemotherapy and radiation.[4,7] In the case of DLGGs, extensive cytoreductive surgery with removal of the anaplastic foci can delay malignant transformation, hence altering the natural history.[2,3,8] For both low-grade and high-grade gliomas, a gross total resection is associated with longer survival and improved neurologic outcomes.[3,9]

As would be expected, studies have shown that maximal resection had more benefit compared with partial resection or biopsy.[10,11] Sanai and colleagues conducted a literature search regarding extent of resection (EOR) and outcomes; for low-grade gliomas, the mean survival improved from 61.1 months to 90.5 months with a greater EOR. In high-grade gliomas, the improvement was from 64.9 to 75.2 months in World Health Organization (WHO) Grade III gliomas and 11.3 to 14.2 months in WHO grade IV gliomas.[9] Brown and colleagues[12] had similar results and concluded that patients with newly diagnosed GBMs who underwent a gross total resection were 61% more likely to survive 1 year, 19% more likely to survive 2 years and 51% more likely to be progression free at 1 year compared with those who had subtotal resection. In regard to EOR, ranges from 78% to 98% have been shown to provide a survival benefit.[13,14]

There remains a balance to be struck between achieving a gross total resection and preventing any new neurologic deficits. Associated technology such as intraoperative MRI, use of fluorescent 5-aminolevulinic acid, artificial intelligence, virtual/augmented reality, and more recently connectomics have improved prospects of maximal safe resection.[4,15–20] Beyond the EOR, the adjunct of standard chemotherapy and radiotherapy, that is, Stupp protocol, for GBMs, can provide a significant survival benefit.[7]

There can be microscopic residual tumor beyond the contrast enhancement and so, a significant chance of recurrence despite near 100% resection of visual tumor.[12,21] Stemming from the records of Dandy, who performed a hemispherectomy for tumor resection of low-grade gliomas in hopes to irradicate all tumor contents, the concept of supramaximal resection has gained momentum.[22] Beyond just resection of the contrast-enhancing tumor, it has been found that resection of the areas with abnormal Fluid-Attenuated Inversion Recovery (FLAIR) and T2 noncontrast enhancement surrounding the contrast-enhanced tumor is associated with improved outcomes.[23–26]

Vivas-Buitrago and colleagues conducted a study looking at 101 patients with newly diagnosed GBMs who underwent resection of their tumors. They found that supramaximal resection (SMR) was associated with improved overall survival in patients with Isocitrate Dehydrogenase (IDH)-wildtype GBMs compared with patients who underwent just gross total resection, however, that finding was true for 20% Supramaximal resection (SMR) and there was no significant effect on overall survival when that percentage exceeded 60%.[27] Although resection of T2 FLAIR hyperintense region surrounding the tumor is likely to contain microscopic infiltrative tumor cells, it also contains functional brain parenchyma. Therefore, it can be challenging to find a balance between maximal diffuse tumor resection and preservation of "normal" functional brain parenchyma. One feasible solution proposed by this group included awake craniotomies with cortical and subcortical mapping and neuropsychological testing when feasible based on tumor location and symptomology. Although the concept of supramaximal resection is believed to lead to better outcomes from the tumor burden standpoint, it is important to consider and balance this with preservation of neurologic function and minimize development of new neurologic deficits.[28]

RADIOFREQUENCY ABLATION FOR INTRACRANIAL TUMORS/GLIOMA

Several minimally invasive techniques were introduced in efforts to achieve the cytoreductive effects of surgery without the associated, morbid complications. These include laser, cryotherapy, radiofrequency microwaves, and focused ultrasound.[29] Radiofrequency ablation is a thermal ablation method which delivers electromagnetic radiation to heat tissue leading to coagulative necrosis.[30] It could be used to treat deep-seated intracranial tumors and could be coupled with MR imaging.[31] It also has the ability to initiate a cell-mediated immune response against the tumor cells, producing a long-term immunity. Some disadvantages include formation of vascular thrombosis, dependence on electrical and thermal tissue conductivity, subject to "heat sink" effect when near vascular structures thus sparing cancer cells close to those blood vessels and formation of a hypoxic microenvironment which could promote tumor progression. Anzai and colleagues[32] found good local control in their 14 primary and metastatic brain tumors treated with radiofrequency ablation.

ADVANTAGES OF LASER-INDUCED THERMAL THERAPY

LITT has evolved over the past two decades as a minimally invasive technique that allows for thermal ablation of several intracranial tumors. Although its uses were initially limited and met with much skepticism, it has gained popularity over the years as it proved its efficacy and safety for several intracranial pathologies. One of the most common uses for LITT today is high-grade gliomas—both newly diagnosed and recurrent. Some of the key characteristics that allowed LITT to grow popular among the neurosurgery world include its efficacy in achieving similar cytoreduction of tumors as does standard surgical resection and allowing for real-time monitoring of tumor ablation, hence minimizing damage to nearby eloquent areas and lowering risk of developing new neurologic deficits.

Some studies suggested a benefit of LITT over surgical resection when treating deep-seated tumors. Barnett and colleagues[33] conducted a systematic review and meta-analysis specifically for high gliomas in or near eloquent area of the brain. Their extent of ablation (EOA) was 85.4% with LITT compared with an EOR of 77% with open craniotomy. In addition, the complication rate was lower for LITT compared with open craniotomy—5.7% versus 13.8%. There was a statistically significant improvement in EOR/EOA and a reduction in major neurocognitive complications with LITT compared with craniotomy. Specifically for high-grade tumors in eloquent brain regions, which are otherwise deemed inoperable or if surgery is offered, it is often limited to just open biopsy or partial resection, LITT provides an acceptable alternative with benefits that are comparable, if not, superior, to those of surgical resection.

Di and colleagues calculated the EOA achieved in their series of 20 patients who underwent LITT for newly diagnosed glioblastomas. They found that in patients with greater than 70% EOA, there was significantly improved progression-free survival (PFS) and a trend toward improved overall survival. PFS was further improved when LITT was followed by early chemotherapy compared with delayed treatments.[34] A study conducted by de Groot and colleagues[35] concluded that median overall survival after LITT with subsequent chemotherapy and radiation was similar to those who had surgical resections.

Mohammadi and colleagues[36] assessed the EOA in 24 patients who underwent LITT for recurrent and newly diagnosed high-grade gliomas. They found that with greater extent of tumor coverage with laser ablation, as defined by tumor damage threshold lines, there was improved PFS. They concluded that the cytoreductive effect of hyperthermia via laser ablation was equivalent to that from surgical debulking. Similarly, Shah and colleagues[37] reported a statistically significant difference in local control when patients underwent greater than 85% EOA compared with ≤85% EOA. Their time to recurrence was 56 months in the greater than 85% EOA group compared with 12.3 months in the ≤85% group. They demonstrated that EOA was the strongest predictor of local control and greater EOA correlated with better local control for multiple types of lesions. As previously mentioned, LITT may show superiority as a treatment option for deep-seated tumors or those in areas of eloquence, when compared with open resection.[33] Although the results of these studies are interesting, it must be noted that open surgery and LITT do carry an inherent difference—the physical cytoreduction with surgery versus the ablative cytoreduction with LITT. The significance of this difference seemed intuitive in the past; however, as more studies have surfaced, it ultimately brings this question back into the spotlight.

A feature of LITT that sets it apart from other techniques and contributed to its appeal is real-time thermal monitoring. McNichols and colleagues described a computer-controlled laser thermal therapy system, which they used to produce lesions in canine and porcine brains and used MRI-based feedback to control the thermal energy and laser ablation.[38] This system was effective in regulating heat, eliminating carbonization and vaporization, and protecting the fiber optic applicators of the lasers. Ultimately, the MRI estimation of thermal dose correlated with thermal necrosis as seen in histologic evaluation. The compatibility of LITT with real-time MRI thermometry allows for safety and quality control thus adding to the efficacy of the procedure for treating intracranial lesions.[39–41]

Other benefits of LITT include ability to use multiple times without concerns for developing dose toxicity, as with radiation, or resistance, as with chemotherapy, patients tend to have shorter hospital stays compared with open craniotomies with faster recoveries and also increased permeability of therapeutic drugs due to disruption of the blood brain barrier (BBB).[1,42–44] Muir and colleagues[45] published their cohort of patients who underwent LITT multiple times for recurrent GBMs and found that the patients tolerated the procedure well and also had a meaningful survival considering the procedure was used as a salvage treatment.

LASER-INDUCED THERMAL THERAPY FOR GLIOMA
Laser-Induced Thermal Therapy for Recurrent Gliomas

Although LITT has been proposed for multiple uses intracranially, a common use is for malignant glioma. Initially, LITT was reserved for tumors that were deemed surgically inoperable or recurrent despite having exhausted more traditional treatment methods. LITT has its own unique benefits for the treatment of recurrent gliomas. Recurrent disease is often focal and smaller as it is often found during more frequent surveillance and therefore is particularly amenable to laser ablation.[44] In addition, repeat surgery in a potentially already frail patient can lead to morbidity and wound healing issues due to prior chemotherapy and radiation. Last, salvage chemotherapy may be more effective following laser ablation.

Compared with newly diagnosed gliomas, recurrent gliomas are particular tougher to treat and have a grim prognosis. Factors found to be associated with poor postoperative survival in patients with recurrent GBMs included tumor location in eloquent brain regions, Karnofsky performance status $\leq$ 80, and tumor volume $\geq$50 cm^3.[46] Often times, at the time of recurrence, many patients are not as healthy to tolerate further open surgery. In fact, only about one of four patients with recurrent GBMs is candidates for reoperation.[47] Especially in those instances, LITT offers a safer alternative that can still decrease tumor burden offering comparable cytoreductive effects through ablation. Multiple studies have shown its efficacy and safety in its use for recurrent gliomas.[48–56]

Treatment with chemotherapy, whether that is monotherapy or combination chemotherapeutic drugs, has been studied as a potential treatment option for recurrent high-grade glioma. Food and Drug Administration (FDA) FDA-approved chemotherapeutic agents for recurrent high-grade gliomas are temozolomide, bevacizumab, lomustine, and carmustine (intravenous or wafer implants), as either single-drug treatment or in combination with other chemotherapeutic drugs, although no single regimen has proven to be superior to others for the treatment of recurrent of progressive glioblastoma.[47,57] Although no studies have directly compared the efficacy of LITT versus any chemotherapeutic regimens, individual studies have shown comparable, if not superior, results of LITT to those of chemotherapy. In a study looking at the use of lomustine and bevacizumab for recurrent glioblastoma, the overall survival was 9.1 months for the drug combination and 8.6 months when lomustine was used alone (P > .05) and PFS was 4.2 months in the combination group and 1.5 months in the single therapy group.[58] This can be compared with an overall survival of 11.6 months seen after 41 recurrent GBMs were treated with LITT.[56] A pooled analysis of all available literature in which LITT was used to treat recurrent GBMs, the authors found a pool overall survival of 18.6 months, a pooled post-LITT survival of 10.2 months and a pooled PFS of 6.2 months.[51] These values suggest that LITT may be favorable to chemotherapy for the treatment of recurrent, progressive glioblastomas.

Laser-Induced Thermal Therapy for Newly Diagnosed Gliomas

LITT is often referred to as a salvage treatment option for recurrent gliomas that have been previously resected and exhausted adjuvant radiation and chemotherapy. However, more recently, neurosurgeons have started to offer this approach for newly diagnosed glioma as well.[48] This approach has been especially offered for gliomas which are deemed surgically inoperable due to deep-seated locations or being near eloquent regions of the brain or for patients who are deemed poor candidates for open surgery due to comorbidities or old age.[44] Some of the tumor locations ideal for upfront LITT therapy include the deep gray matter structures such as thalamus and basal ganglia, corpus callosum, or insula.

Ivan and colleagues showed their early results of 25 patients who underwent laser ablation for newly diagnosed glioma. Their cohort had a mean overall survival of 14.2 month and a complication rate of 3.4%.[59] Similarly, Muir and colleagues[60] presented their series of 20 patients with newly diagnosed, "inoperable" GBMs and concluded that those patients had similar survival times and local recurrence rates as patients who underwent surgical resection.

LITT seems to be a growing option for surgically inaccessible, deep-seated lesions such as those near the brainstem or deeper gray matter regions.[61] Shah and colleagues[62] had a mean EOA of 98.5% and mean PFS of 14.3 months in their cohort of 74 patients who underwent LITT for deep-seated gliomas that were deemed surgically inaccessible. Ashraf and colleagues[63] presented a multi-institutional study reviewing the results of LITT for lesions within the posterior fossa. It was noted that the lesions tended to be smaller in size compared with their supratentorial counterparts. The complication rate was approximately 24% and it was advised that extra caution must be taken to prevent damage to surrounding neural structures as there is relatively more surrounding eloquent tissue in the posterior fossa compared with the supratentorial space. Dadey and colleagues[64] further demonstrated the importance of precise and accurate placement of the laser probe using stereotactic guidance to ensure effective ablation of these deep-seated lesions without major complications. Other studies also supported LITT as an effective option for posterior fossa tumors.[65,66]

THE ROLE OF LASER-INDUCED THERMAL THERAPY IN DISRUPTION OF THE BLOOD BRAIN BARRIER

As noted earlier, LITT has been shown to increase permeability of therapeutic drugs due to disruption of the BBB. This may make it useful in salvage cases as adjuvant chemotherapy may be more effective following laser ablation. The BBB presents a unique obstacle in the physiology and treatment of intracranial brain tumors, compared with lesions elsewhere in the body. A variety of specialized cell types including endothelial cells, astrocytes, pericytes, microglia and neuron function together to regulate selective permeability and cellular transport, hence regulating homeostasis as well as cerebral blood flow. This vigilant regulation further restricts the targeted delivery of therapeutic drugs for the treatment of high-grade gliomas.[67]

Furthermore, high-grade gliomas and intracranial metastases also have the ability to generate a blood-tumor barrier (BTB). Through angiogenesis and neovascularization, a hallmark characteristic of GBMs, the tumors develop immature, dilated, and leaky vessels. These create a high interstitial pressure within the tumor itself and lead to a more malignant phenotype of tumors. In fact, the BTB is more permeable in the core of the tumor compared with the periphery and the BBB distinguishing the tumor from the normal brain parenchyma is impermeable. These characteristics allow for the malignant, aggressive nature of these high-grade tumors while also creating a barrier from the normal brain matter and vasculature to prevent any therapeutic agents to enter.[67]

In the past, some of the therapeutic methods used to try to overcome these obstacles included intrathecal delivery of chemotherapy drugs through Ommaya reservoirs and direct delivery to the tumor itself using chemotherapeutic wafers.[67–72] Bregy and colleagues[73] did a literature search yielding a total of 19 studies and 795 patients who underwent glial wafer implantation. It was found that the mean overall survival time increased from 14 months to 16.2 months when Gliadel wafers were added on to standard treatment of surgery, radiation and systemic chemotherapy. Overall, although these wafers did marginally increase survival and local control, they were associated with a high complication rate, up to 42.7% in their cohort. For this reason, the group recommended against using gliadel wafers.[43,74–78]

The idea that hyperthermia can treat malignancy has been around for some time and body hyperthermia was indeed used as a means to disrupt the BBB and allow entrance of chemotherapeutic agents. However, as these methods were systemic, there was the risk of causing damage to other parts of the body as well.[67,79] This brought about the concept of targeted hyperthermia in hopes to directly provide thermal energy to the tumor site, disrupting the BBB and BTB and also treating the tumor cells themselves. In as early as the 1980s, studies were conducted in which microwave radiator/sensors were implanted into the site of GBMs or high-grade astrocytomas.[80,81]

The use of lasers to provide hyperthermia to tissues had been seen for many years prior. Although ruby and CO_2, lasers had been used previously for the treatment of tumors, it was the introduction of the neodymium-doped yttrium aluminum garnet (Nd-YAG) lasers that would lead to what we currently use today for laser ablation of intracranial tumors.[82,83]

Salehi and colleagues[84] used a mouse model to demonstrate the effects of LITT on the BBB and BTB and found that there was local disruption of the BBB and BTB leading to increased permeability for up to 30 days following the procedure. Specifically, the therapy decreased the integrity of the tight junctions of this molecular barrier and increased endothelial cell transcytosis. This, then, allows large molecules including human immunoglobulins to pass through the targeted area. In the mouse model, laser ablation and adjuvant chemotherapy with doxorubicin, which is normally not permeable across the BBB, led to increased survival.

Leuthardt and colleagues[43] calculated the degree and timing of BBB disruption following laser ablation in patients with recurrent GBM.

Specifically, they calculated the vascular transfer constant as an indicator of permeability as well as serum levels of neuron-specific enolase. They found that based on the values and their trends following laser ablation, there was a peak of highest permeability of the BBB, within 1 to 2 weeks of laser ablation, which declined and resolved within 4 to 6 weeks. This in turn suggested a therapeutic window during which administering earlier adjuvant chemotherapy may have maximal benefits for these patients. Multiple clinical trials are underway, showing the benefits of different chemotherapy regimens and their efficacy when used in conjunction with LITT.[85–87]

SUMMARY

LITT has evolved over the past decade and proved its efficacy and safety for the treatment of a variety of intracranial pathologies, including gliomas. From being used solely as a salvage treatment of recurrent gliomas, it now is often used first line for certain newly diagnosed gliomas. It is comparable to the standard treatment of surgical resection in allowing maximal ablative cytoreduction while minimizing damage to surrounding eloquent brain matter and thus improved overall and PFS while maintaining a relatively low complication rate. As neurosurgeons gain more experience with the technique, it is believed that LITT will continue to progress as a first-line cytoreductive treatment for a number of intracranial pathologies.

CLINICS CARE POINTS

- Maximal resection/ablation is associated with better outcomes in patients with high grade gliomas.
- Laser ablation shows superiority over open resection for the treatment of deep-seated, "surgically inoperable"
- LITT may enhance the effects of chemotherapeutic agents by increasing blood brain barrier permeability.

DISCLOSURES

None of the authors above have any financial disclosures to report.

REFERENCES

1. Patel P, Patel NV, Danish SF. Intracranial MR-guided laser-induced thermal therapy: single-center experience with the Visualase thermal therapy system. J Neurosurg 2016;1–8. https://doi.org/10.3171/2015.7.JNS15244.
2. Smits A, Jakola AS. Clinical presentation, natural history, and prognosis of diffuse low-grade gliomas. Neurosurg Clin N Am 2019;30(1):35–42.
3. DeAngelis LM. Brain tumors. N Engl J Med 2001;344(2):114–23.
4. Wen PY, Weller M, Lee EQ, et al. Glioblastoma in adults: a Society for Neuro-Oncology (SNO) and European Society of Neuro-Oncology (EANO) consensus review on current management and future directions. Neuro Oncol 2020;22(8):1073–113.
5. Berger TR, Wen PY, Lang-Orsini M, et al. World Health Organization 2021 classification of central nervous system tumors and implications for therapy for adult-type gliomas: a review. JAMA Oncol 2022;8(10):1493–501.
6. Louis DN, Perry A, Wesseling P, et al. The 2021 WHO classification of tumors of the central nervous system: a summary. Neuro Oncol 2021;23(8):1231–51.
7. Stupp R, Mason WP, van den Bent MJ, et al. Radiotherapy plus concomitant and adjuvant temozolomide for glioblastoma. N Engl J Med 2005;352(10):987–96.
8. Jakola AS, Myrmel KS, Kloster R, et al. Comparison of a strategy favoring early surgical resection vs a strategy favoring watchful waiting in low-grade gliomas. JAMA 2012;308(18):1881–8.
9. Sanai N, Berger MS. Glioma extent of resection and its impact on patient outcome. Neurosurgery 2008;62(4):753–64 [discussion: 264–6].
10. Stummer W, Reulen HJ, Meinel T, et al. Extent of resection and survival in glioblastoma multiforme: identification of and adjustment for bias. Neurosurgery 2008;62(3):564–76 [discussion: 564–76].
11. Vuorinen V, Hinkka S, Farkkila M, et al. Debulking or biopsy of malignant glioma in elderly people - a randomised study. Acta Neurochir (Wien) 2003;145(1):5–10.
12. Brown TJ, Brennan MC, Li M, et al. Association of the extent of resection with survival in glioblastoma: a systematic review and meta-analysis. JAMA Oncol 2016;2(11):1460–9.
13. Lacroix M, Abi-Said D, Fourney DR, et al. A multivariate analysis of 416 patients with glioblastoma multiforme: prognosis, extent of resection, and survival. J Neurosurg 2001;95(2):190–8.
14. Sanai N, Polley MY, McDermott MW, et al. An extent of resection threshold for newly diagnosed glioblastomas. J Neurosurg 2011;115(1):3–8.
15. Hardesty DA, Sanai N. The value of glioma extent of resection in the modern neurosurgical era. Front Neurol 2012;3:140.
16. Stummer W, Pichlmeier U, Meinel T, et al. Fluorescence-guided surgery with 5-aminolevulinic acid for resection of malignant glioma: a randomised

controlled multicentre phase III trial. Lancet Oncol 2006;7(5):392–401.

17. Eatz TA, Eichberg DG, Lu VM, et al. Intraoperative 5-ALA fluorescence-guided resection of high-grade glioma leads to greater extent of resection with better outcomes: a systematic review. J Neurooncol 2022;156(2):233–56.

18. Satoh M, Nakajima T, Yamaguchi T, et al. Evaluation of augmented-reality based navigation for brain tumor surgery. J Clin Neurosci 2021;94:305–14.

19. Henderson F, Abdullah KG, Verma R, et al. Tractography and the connectome in neurosurgical treatment of gliomas: the premise, the progress, and the potential. Neurosurg Focus 2020;48(2):E6.

20. Duffau H. Brain connectomics applied to oncological neuroscience: from a traditional surgical strategy focusing on glioma topography to a meta-network approach. Acta Neurochir (Wien) 2021;163(4):905–17.

21. Hirono S, Ozaki K, Kobayashi M, et al. Oncological and functional outcomes of supratotal resection of IDH1 wild-type glioblastoma based on (11)C-methionine PET: a retrospective, single-center study. Sci Rep 2021;11(1):14554.

22. Bell E Jr, Karnosh LJ. Cerebral hemispherectomy; report of a case 10 years after operation. J Neurosurg 1949;6(4):285–93.

23. Li YM, Suki D, Hess K, et al. The influence of maximum safe resection of glioblastoma on survival in 1229 patients: can we do better than gross-total resection? J Neurosurg 2016;124(4):977–88.

24. de Leeuw CN, Vogelbaum MA. Supratotal resection in glioma: a systematic review. Neuro Oncol 2019; 21(2):179–88.

25. D'Amico RS, Englander ZK, Canoll P, et al. Extent of resection in glioma-a review of the cutting edge. World Neurosurg 2017;103:538–49.

26. Smith JS, Chang EF, Lamborn KR, et al. Role of extent of resection in the long-term outcome of low-grade hemispheric gliomas. J Clin Oncol 2008; 26(8):1338–45.

27. Vivas-Buitrago T, Domingo RA, Tripathi S, et al. Influence of supramarginal resection on survival outcomes after gross-total resection of IDH-wild-type glioblastoma. J Neurosurg 2022;136(1):1–8.

28. Guerrini F, Roca E, Spena G. Supramarginal resection for glioblastoma: it is time to set boundaries! A critical review on a hot topic. Brain Sci 2022;(5): 12. https://doi.org/10.3390/brainsci12050652.

29. Merkle EM, Shonk JR, Zheng L, et al. MR imaging-guided radiofrequency thermal ablation in the porcine brain at 0.2 T. Eur Radiol 2001;11(5):884–92.

30. Partridge B, Rossmeisl JH, Kaloss AM, et al. Novel ablation methods for treatment of gliomas. J Neurosci Methods 2020;336:108630.

31. Franzini A, Moosa S, Servello D, et al. Ablative brain surgery: an overview. Int J Hyperthermia 2019;36(2): 64–80.

32. Anzai Y, Lufkin R, DeSalles A, et al. Preliminary experience with MR-guided thermal ablation of brain tumors. AJNR Am J Neuroradiol 1995;16(1):39–48 [discussion: 49–52].

33. Barnett GH, Voigt JD, Alhuwalia MS. A systematic review and meta-analysis of studies examining the use of brain laser interstitial thermal therapy versus craniotomy for the treatment of high-grade tumors in or near areas of eloquence: an examination of the extent of resection and major complication rates associated with each type of surgery. Stereotact Funct Neurosurg 2016;94(3):164–73.

34. Di L, Wang CP, Shah AH, et al. A cohort study on prognostic factors for laser interstitial thermal therapy success in newly diagnosed glioblastoma. Neurosurgery 2021;89(3):496–503.

35. de Groot JF, Kim AH, Prabhu S, et al. Efficacy of laser interstitial thermal therapy (LITT) for newly diagnosed and recurrent IDH wild-type glioblastoma. Neurooncol Adv 2022;4(1):vdac040.

36. Mohammadi AM, Hawasli AH, Rodriguez A, et al. The role of laser interstitial thermal therapy in enhancing progression-free survival of difficult-to-access high-grade gliomas: a multicenter study. Cancer Med 2014;3(4):971–9.

37. Shah AH, Semonche A, Eichberg DG, et al. The role of laser interstitial thermal therapy in surgical neuro-oncology: series of 100 consecutive patients. Neurosurgery 2020;87(2):266–75.

38. McNichols RJ, Gowda A, Kangasniemi M, et al. MR thermometry-based feedback control of laser interstitial thermal therapy at 980 nm. Lasers Surg Med 2004;34(1):48–55.

39. Carpentier A, McNichols RJ, Stafford RJ, et al. Laser thermal therapy: real-time MRI-guided and computer-controlled procedures for metastatic brain tumors. Lasers Surg Med 2011;43(10):943–50.

40. Carpentier A, McNichols RJ, Stafford RJ, et al. Real-time magnetic resonance-guided laser thermal therapy for focal metastatic brain tumors. Neurosurgery 2008;63(1 Suppl 1):ONS21–8 [discussion: ONS28–9].

41. Missios S, Bekelis K, Barnett GH. Renaissance of laser interstitial thermal ablation. Neurosurg Focus 2015;38(3):E13.

42. Viozzi I, Guberinic A, Overduin CG, et al. Laser interstitial thermal therapy in patients with newly diagnosed glioblastoma: a systematic review. J Clin Med 2021;(2):10. https://doi.org/10.3390/jcm100 20355.

43. Leuthardt EC, Duan C, Kim MJ, et al. Hyperthermic laser ablation of recurrent glioblastoma leads to temporary disruption of the peritumoral blood brain barrier. PLoS One 2016;11(2):e0148613.

44. Hawasli AH, Kim AH, Dunn GP, et al. Stereotactic laser ablation of high-grade gliomas. Neurosurg Focus 2014;37(6):E1.

45. Muir M, Traylor JI, Gadot R, et al. Repeat laser interstitial thermal therapy for recurrent primary and metastatic intracranial tumors. Surg Neurol Int 2022;13: 311.

46. Park JK, Hodges T, Arko L, et al. Scale to predict survival after surgery for recurrent glioblastoma multiforme. J Clin Oncol 2010;28(24):3838–43.

47. Weller M, Cloughesy T, Perry JR, et al. Standards of care for treatment of recurrent glioblastoma–are we there yet? Neuro Oncol 2013;15(1):4–27.

48. Thomas JG, Rao G, Kew Y, et al. Laser interstitial thermal therapy for newly diagnosed and recurrent glioblastoma. Neurosurg Focus 2016;41(4):E12.

49. Lee I, Kalkanis S, Hadjipanayis CG. Stereotactic laser interstitial thermal therapy for recurrent high-grade gliomas. Neurosurgery 2016;79(Suppl 1): S24–34.

50. Rodriguez A, Tatter SB. Laser ablation of recurrent malignant gliomas: current status and future perspective. Neurosurgery 2016;79(Suppl 1):S35–9.

51. Munoz-Casabella A, Alvi MA, Rahman M, et al. Laser interstitial thermal therapy for recurrent glioblastoma: pooled analyses of available literature. World Neurosurg 2021;153:91–7.e1.

52. Schwarzmaier HJ, Eickmeyer F, von Tempelhoff W, et al. MR-guided laser-induced interstitial thermotherapy of recurrent glioblastoma multiforme: preliminary results in 16 patients. Eur J Radiol 2006;59(2): 208–15.

53. Sloan AE, Ahluwalia MS, Valerio-Pascua J, et al. Results of the NeuroBlate system first-in-humans Phase I clinical trial for recurrent glioblastoma: clinical article. J Neurosurg 2013;118(6):1202–19.

54. Carpentier A, Chauvet D, Reina V, et al. MR-guided laser-induced thermal therapy (LITT) for recurrent glioblastomas. Lasers Surg Med 2012;44(5):361–8.

55. Montemurro N, Anania Y, Cagnazzo F, et al. Survival outcomes in patients with recurrent glioblastoma treated with Laser Interstitial Thermal Therapy (LITT): a systematic review. Clin Neurol Neurosurg 2020;195:105942.

56. Kamath AA, Friedman DD, Akbari SHA, et al. Glioblastoma treated with magnetic resonance imaging-guided laser interstitial thermal therapy: safety, efficacy, and outcomes. Neurosurgery 2019; 84(4):836–43.

57. Fisher JP, Adamson DC. Current FDA-approved therapies for high-grade malignant gliomas. Biomedicines 2021;(3):9. https://doi.org/10.3390/bio medicines9030324.

58. Wick W, Gorlia T, Bendszus M, et al. Lomustine and bevacizumab in progressive glioblastoma. N Engl J Med 2017;377(20):1954–63.

59. Ivan ME, Mohammadi AM, De Deugd N, et al. Laser ablation of newly diagnosed malignant gliomas: a meta-analysis. Neurosurgery 2016;79(Suppl 1): S17–23.

60. Muir M, Patel R, Traylor JI, et al. Laser interstitial thermal therapy for newly diagnosed glioblastoma. Lasers Med Sci 2022;37(3):1811–20.

61. Silva D, Sharma M, Barnett GH. Laser ablation vs open resection for deep-seated tumors: evidence for laser ablation. Neurosurgery 2016;63(Suppl 1): 15–26.

62. Shah AH, Burks JD, Buttrick SS, et al. Laser interstitial thermal therapy as a primary treatment for deep inaccessible gliomas. Neurosurgery 2019;84(3): 768–77.

63. Ashraf O, Arzumanov G, Luther E, et al. Magnetic resonance-guided laser interstitial thermal therapy for posterior fossa neoplasms. J Neurooncol 2020; 149(3):533–42.

64. Dadey DY, Kamath AA, Smyth MD, et al. Utilizing personalized stereotactic frames for laser interstitial thermal ablation of posterior fossa and mesiotemporal brain lesions: a single-institution series. Neurosurg Focus 2016;41(4):E4.

65. Borghei-Razavi H, Koech H, Sharma M, et al. Laser interstitial thermal therapy for posterior fossa lesions: an initial experience. World Neurosurg 2018; 117:e146–53.

66. Sabahi M, Bordes SJ, Najera E, et al. Laser interstitial thermal therapy for posterior fossa lesions: a systematic review and analysis of multi-institutional outcomes. Cancers (Basel) 2022;14(2). https://doi. org/10.3390/cancers14020456.

67. Patel B, Yang PH, Kim AH. The effect of thermal therapy on the blood-brain barrier and blood-tumor barrier. Int J Hyperthermia 2020;37(2):35–43.

68. Kennedy BC, Brown LT, Komotar RJ, et al. Stereotactic catheter placement for Ommaya reservoirs. J Clin Neurosci 2016;27:44–7.

69. Sandberg DI, Bilsky MH, Souweidane MM, et al. Ommaya reservoirs for the treatment of leptomeningeal metastases. Neurosurgery 2000;47(1):49–54 [discussion: 54–5].

70. Hart MG, Grant R, Garside R, et al. Chemotherapeutic wafers for high grade glioma. Cochrane Database Syst Rev 2008;(3):CD007294.

71. Perry J, Chambers A, Spithoff K, et al. Gliadel wafers in the treatment of malignant glioma: a systematic review. Curr Oncol 2007;14(5):189–94.

72. Ashby LS, Smith KA, Stea B. Gliadel wafer implantation combined with standard radiotherapy and concurrent followed by adjuvant temozolomide for treatment of newly diagnosed high-grade glioma: a systematic literature review. World J Surg Oncol 2016;14(1):225.

73. Bregy A, Shah AH, Diaz MV, et al. The role of Gliadel wafers in the treatment of high-grade gliomas. Expert Rev Anticancer Ther 2013;13(12):1453–61.

74. Westphal M, Ram Z, Riddle V, et al, Executive Committee of the Gliadel Study G. Gliadel wafer in initial surgery for malignant glioma: long-term follow-up of

a multicenter controlled trial. Acta Neurochir (Wien) 2006;148(3):269–75 [discussion: 275].

75. Westphal M, Hilt DC, Bortey E, et al. A phase 3 trial of local chemotherapy with biodegradable carmustine (BCNU) wafers (Gliadel wafers) in patients with primary malignant glioma. Neuro Oncol 2003; 5(2):79–88.

76. Nagpal S. The role of BCNU polymer wafers (Gliadel) in the treatment of malignant glioma. Neurosurg Clin N Am 2012;23(2):289–95, ix.

77. Brem H, Piantadosi S, Burger PC, et al. Placebo-controlled trial of safety and efficacy of intraoperative controlled delivery by biodegradable polymers of chemotherapy for recurrent gliomas. The Polymer-brain Tumor Treatment Group. Lancet 1995;345(8956):1008–12.

78. Attenello FJ, Mukherjee D, Datoo G, et al. Use of Gliadel (BCNU) wafer in the surgical treatment of malignant glioma: a 10-year institutional experience. Ann Surg Oncol 2008;15(10):2887–93.

79. Salcman M, Samaras GM. Hyperthermia for brain tumors: biophysical rationale. Neurosurgery 1981; 9(3):327–35.

80. Salcman M, Samaras GM. Interstitial microwave hyperthermia for brain tumors. Results of a phase-1 clinical trial. J Neurooncol 1983;1(3):225–36.

81. Stea B, Cetas TC, Cassady JR, et al. Interstitial thermoradiotherapy of brain tumors: preliminary results of a phase I clinical trial. Int J Radiat Oncol Biol Phys 1990;19(6):1463–71.

82. Schupper AJ, Chanenchuk T, Racanelli A, et al. Laser hyperthermia: past, present, and future. Neuro Oncol 2022;24(Suppl 6):S42–51.

83. Bown SG. Phototherapy in tumors. World J Surg 1983;7(6):700–9.

84. Salehi A, Paturu MR, Patel B, et al. Therapeutic enhancement of blood-brain and blood-tumor barriers permeability by laser interstitial thermal therapy. Neurooncol Adv 2020;2(1):vdaa071.

85. Butt OH, Zhou AY, Huang J, et al. A phase II study of laser interstitial thermal therapy combined with doxorubicin in patients with recurrent glioblastoma. Neurooncol Adv 2021;3(1):vdab164.

86. Hormigo A, Mandeli J, Hadjipanayis C, et al. Phase I study of PD-L1 inhibition with avelumab and laser interstitial thermal therapy in patients with recurrent glioblastoma. J Clin Oncol 2019;37(15).

87. Hwang H, Huang J, Khaddour K, et al. Prolonged response of recurrent IDH-wild-type glioblastoma to laser interstitial thermal therapy with pembrolizumab. CNS Oncol 2022;11(1):CNS81.

Laser Interstitial Thermal Therapy for Radionecrosis

Alexis Paul Romain Terrapon, MD[a], Marie Krüger, MD[a,b,c], Thomas Hundsberger, MD[d], Marian Christoph Neidert, MD[a], Oliver Bozinov, MD[a,*]

KEYWORDS

• Radiation necrosis • LITT • Review • Ablation • Outcome • Safety • Recurrence • Radiotherapy

KEY POINTS

- [For radionecrosis,] laser interstitial thermal therapy (LITT) might be more effective than medical therapy in prolonging survival and may reduce the risk of progression, help taper off steroids, and improve/resolve neurological symptoms.
- Although new imaging modalities exist, radionecrosis remains challenging to diagnose, and although biopsy may help to differentiate lesions it is subject to sampling bias.
- Lesion volume and surrounding edema may increase in the short-/medium-term following LITT, which is not progression but may worsen mass effect: LITT should be used with caution or be avoided in patients with large lesions or acute neurological symptoms.
- Initial increase in edema may require steroid use following LITT, but most patients can be weaned off steroids fast and thus net steroid use is reduced.
- Larger ablation volumes (even supralesional) may improve outcome and should be favored.

INTRODUCTION
Radionecrosis—Background, Definition, Incidence, and Pathophysiology

Brain tumors are usually treated by a combination of surgery, systemic therapy, and radiotherapy, the latter being particularly important in the management of brain metastases. Nowadays, stereotactic radiosurgery is often used as an alternative to whole-brain radiation therapy, in combination with surgery, or as a first-line treatment in nonacute life-threatening oligometastatic disease with lesions under 3 cm.[1] Unfortunately, similar to every treatment option, radiotherapy may cause short- and/or long-term adverse effects. Radiation necrosis (RN) is defined as a severe local tissue reaction occurring at least 3 to 12 months after radiotherapy, with an incidence that varies from 6.5% to 50% according to the modality of radiation, the total dose, the fractionation, the underlying pathology, and diagnostic methodology.[2] This incidence is documented between 14% and 15% for conventional modalities, between 4.7% and 9.2% for stereotactic radiosurgery for brain metastases, and up to 22.6% for large lesions (also stereotactic radiosurgery) or even 50% following brachytherapy.[2] Although the pathophysiology of RN is currently not completely understood, it is believed to be the result of a combination of initial vascular insult and subsequent brain parenchymal injury.[2] Both changes cause endothelial, microglial, neural, and tumoral cell damage, which produces reactive oxygen species and promotes apoptosis, fibrinoid necrosis, blood-brain barrier disruption, cerebral edema, and demyelination.

[a] Department of Neurosurgery, Kantonsspital St. Gallen, Medical School St. Gallen, Rorschacher Strasse 95, St. Gallen 9007, Switzerland; [b] Unit of Functional Neurosurgery, Institute of Neurology and Neurosurgery, 33 Queen Square, London WC1N 3BG, UK; [c] Department of Stereotactic and Functional Neurosurgery, University Medical Center Freiburg, Breisacher Strasse 64, Freiburg 79095, Germany; [d] Department of Neurology and of Oncology, Kantonsspital St. Gallen, Medical School St. Gallen, Rorschacher Strasse 95, St. Gallen 9007, Switzerland
* Corresponding author. Chefarzt, Klinik für Neurochirurgie, Rorschacher Strasse 95, St. Gallen 9007, Switzerland.
E-mail address: oliver.bozinov@kssg.ch

Neurosurg Clin N Am 34 (2023) 209–225
https://doi.org/10.1016/j.nec.2022.11.001
1042-3680/23/© 2022 Elsevier Inc. All rights reserved.

Evaluation of Radionecrosis and Challenges

Patients suffering from RN may present with mild-to-severe cognitive and/or neurological deficits, symptoms of increased intracranial pressure, seizures, and rarely cerebral hemorrhage.[2,3] MRI features of RN include an increase in T2- fluid-attenuated inversion recovery (FLAIR) signal corresponding to edema, contrast leakage to surrounding normal brain tissue, decrease in regional cerebral blood volume, and increase in apparent diffusion coefficient.[3] Unfortunately, clinical presentation and radiological features of RN and tumor recurrence or progression following radiotherapy mostly overlap, which greatly complicates their distinction; this is a severe drawback for decision-making, given their contrasting treatment and prognosis. New imaging modalities such as magnetic resonance perfusion, magnetic resonance spectroscopy, PET, and single-photon emission computed tomography improve diagnostic accuracy but can be costly. Despite surgical risks and sampling bias, biopsy is still considered safe to confirm an RN.[2,4] An additional concern is that lesions following radiotherapy are often a combination of tumor cells and radiation injury, which complicates their classification/therapy and greatly increases the risk of sample bias. Recent recommendations aim to review as many characteristics as possible to identify the predominant component of the lesion instead of considering both mechanisms as complete separate entities.[3]

Therapeutic Options

Conservative treatment options for RN include corticosteroids, bevacizumab, hyperbaric oxygen, and anticoagulants.[5,6] Steroids can often rapidly improve symptoms, but they only confer symptomatic relief and may cause side effects or lower the efficacy of immunotherapy.[5] Bevacizumab was shown to improve the clinical symptoms of patients with RN and even to reduce lesion volume but is also associated with severe side effects and high costs.[5,6] For patients in need of urgent treatment or refractory to medical treatment, surgical resection remains of central importance, with the additional benefit of providing tissue samples. However, surgery is invasive, not well suited to deep-seated lesions, and normal brain tissue around the resection cavity may continue to cause necrosis even after complete resection.[6]

Laser Interstitial Thermal Therapy for Radionecrosis

In the last 10 years, laser interstitial thermal therapy (LITT) has increasingly been used to manage RN refractory to medical treatment. Because of its stereotactic precision and minimal invasiveness, LITT may reduce the risk of surgery and enable the targeting of difficult to access lesions by means of open surgery while still providing tissue sample and long-term reduction of edema and lesion volume. In the following article, the authors systematically report and discuss the available evidence relating to LITT for RN.

METHODS

To retrieve all reports of patient outcome following LITT for (suspicion of) RN, the authors conducted a structured literature search on Pubmed on 1st October 2022 with the terms (((radiation) AND (necrosis)) OR (radionecrosis)) AND ((LITT) OR ((laser) AND ((ablation) OR ((thermotherapy) OR ((thermal) AND (therapy)))))) NOT (animals[mesh] NOT humans[mesh]) and retrieved 207 records. They screened all titles/abstracts and/or full-texts and found 32 relevant studies. In addition, references of key articles were screened and 1 supplementary relevant article was found. All full-texts (n = 33) were retrieved, and all studies are summarized in **Table 1**.

RESULTS
Pioneering Studies

The first to describe the use of real-time MR-guided LITT for recurrent brain metastases following chemotherapy, radiotherapy, and radiosurgery were Carpentier and colleagues[7,8] in 2008, but patients with a suspicion of RN were excluded from their study. They published their final results in 2011 with no recurrence within the thermal ablation zone, a median survival of 19.8 months, and no serious adverse event (AE).[9] In 2012, Rahmathulla and colleagues[10] reported the first use of LITT for a biopsy-proven RN refractory to medical treatment in a patient with a history of non–small cell lung cancer with brain metastases treated with stereotactic radiosurgery. The patient, whose symptoms had been resistant to steroids for 6 months, was discharged within 48 hours of surgery and weaned from steroids within 7 weeks, with near complete neurological improvement. At that time, perilesional edema had nearly disappeared despite an increase in lesion size. Rahmathulla and colleagues hypothesized that LITT replaced endothelial proliferating cells and zone of disorganized angiogenesis with thrombosed vessels.

Clinical Outcomes

These results have led to multiple studies describing the use of LITT for RN or recurrent

Table 1
Summary of the available evidence

Authors	Center	Study Type and Purpose	n LITT/n LITT for RN	Progression (only for RN, if NOS)	Survival (only for RN, if NOS)	AE (for all Patients, including other diagnoses than RN, if NOS)	Comments	Lessons
Sankey et al,[34] 2022	• Duke University Medical Center • Cleveland Clinic	• Multicenter retrospective cohort study • LITT vs steroids alone for RN	57/57	Median PFS 13.6 mo	Median survival 15.2 mo	• Scalp burn secondary to drilling (n = 1) • Intraoperative de-saturation leading to procedure prolongation (n = 1) • Seizure within 90 days (n = 7)	—	LITT significantly decreases time to steroid independence for RN following radiation for brain metastases as compared with medical treatment
Riviere-Cazaux et al,[19] 2022	Mayo Clinic: • Rochester • Phoenix • Jacksonville	• Multicenter retrospective • LITT for recurrent metastases/RN	23/13 (only 14 received biopsy)	81.8% with lasting local control until fu (mean fu time unknown)	Median survival 16 mo	• Mild transient language and cognitive/memory change (n = 2) • Left-sided visual loss and word-finding difficulty for 10 minutes (n = 1) • Mild visual symptoms with mild diplopia (n = 1)	Results provided for all cases (no subanalysis for biopsy-proven RN)	LITT was associated with sustained local control in most of the patients treated for radiographic progression after radiation of central metastases
Luther et al,[28] 2021	University of Miami Miller School of Medicine	• Single-center retrospective • Outcome for different LITT volumes for posterior fossa lesions	17/5	—	—	• Transient neurological deficits (n = 2)	No separate results for RN	Patients with radical ablation showed a greater decrease in perilesional edema and an improved functional status immediately and at last follow-up

(continued on next page)

Table 1
(continued)

Authors	Center	Study Type and Purpose	n LITT/n LITT for RN	Progression (only for RN, if NOS)	Survival (only for RN, if NOS)	AE (for all Patients, including other diagnoses than RN, if NOS)	Comments	Lessons
Lanier et al,[23] 2021	Wake Forest School of Medicine	• Single-center retrospective • Outcome of LITT for RN	30/30	• 3 mo: 95.7% without progression • 6 mo: 90.9% • 9 mo: 90.9%	Median survival 2.1 years, 18 patients still alive at last fu	• Subacute edema (n = 1) • Intraparenchymal hemorrhage (n = 1)	2 patients with progression within 4 mo of treatment (salvageable)	LITT was safe and durably effective with only 2 recurrences; PRO showed no severe decline and stable well-being and functionality following LITT
Kaye et al,[18] 2020	Rutgers Robert Wood Johnson Medical School	• Single-center retrospective • Influence of LITT on neurological death for in-field recurrence of metastases after radiation	97 (70 patients)/ 97 recurrent metastases or RN	• 7 patients with local recurrence with a median time of 5.6 mo	• 24-mo cumulative incidence of death: 75.4% (36.9% non-neurologic, 30.8% neurologic, 7.7% unknown cause)	• New permanent neurological deficits (n = 3)	• No separate results for RN	Young patients with high baseline KPS and stable systemic disease had the best outcome after LITT
Bastos et al,[39] 2020	University of Texas MD Anderson Cancer Center	• Single-center retrospective • LITT for brain metastases	82 (61 patients)/ 31	Median time to local recurrence not reached at 24 mo	—	• Medical (n =4) • Transient neurological deficits (n = 3) • Persistent neurological deficits (n = 8) • Technical issue with abandon of the procedure (n = 1)	—	Following LITT, tumor recurrence/new tumors had shorter time to recurrence as compared with RN
Ginalis & Danish,[17] 2020	Rutgers Robert Wood Johnson Medical School	• Single-center retrospective • LITT for patients between 65–74 y vs >75 y for intracranial tumors (including RN)	64 (55 patients)/ 40 recurrent metastases or RN	—	• 30-day survival 97.5%	• Inaccurate laser placement (n = 1) • Increased weakness (n =7) • Aphasia (n = 2) • Confusion due to edema (n = 1) • Cognitive deficits (n = 1)	No separate results for RN	LITT was safe for treatment of intracranial tumors and RN in geriatric patients

Study	Institution	Study design	Patients (LITT/total)	PFS	Survival	Complications	RN-specific result	Conclusions
Luther et al,[29] 2020	University of Miami Miller School of Medicine	• Single-center retrospective • Outcome for different LITT volumes for RN	20/20	Mean PFS 5.8 mo	Mean survival 14.3 mo	• Transient altered mental status (n = 1) • Cerebrospinal fluid leak requiring surgical repair (n = 1) • Seizure (n = 1) • Pulmonary embolism (n = 1)	—	Larger ablation volumes (up to >200% of lesion volume) reduced perilesional edema, improved clinical functional status, and did not increase risk
Sujjantarat et al,[33] 2020	Yale University	• Single-center retrospective • LITT vs bevacizumab for RN	25/25	Median PFS 12.1 mo (range 0–64.6 mo)	Median survival 24.8 mo (range 6.0–89.0 mo)	• Confusion (n = 1) • Worsening of left-sided weakness (n = 1) • Seizure and bilateral deep vein thrombosis (n = 1)	—	LITT showed longer overall survival and better long-term lesional volume reduction than bevacizumab
Shah et al,[22] 2020	University of Miami Miller School of Medicine	• Single-center retrospective • Safety and outcome of LITT for intracranial tumors (including RN)	91 patients with 100 LITT/20	25% with recurrence, timing not known	Median survival 16.4 mo	• Transient facial palsy (n = 1) • Post-op seizure (n = 1) • Wound infection (n =2)	No adverse event in the RN group	LITT is safe in surgical neuro-oncology, extent of ablation predicted local control, extent of resection >85% predicted longer PFS (for all cases)
Shao et al,[40] 2020	Cleveland Clinic	• Single-center retrospective • LITT for patients treated before vs after 2014 for intracranial tumors (including RN)	238/50	—	—	• Temporary deficits (n = 68) • Permanent deficits (n = 25) • Seizures (n = 2) • Large hemorrhage (n = 26) • Hemorrhage requiring surgery (n = 3) • Infection (n = 3) • Death within 30 days (n = 6)	No separate results for RN	Efficiency and safety of LITT was improved since 2014

(continued on next page)

Table 1
(continued)

Authors	Center	Study Type and Purpose	n LITT/n LITT for RN	Progression (only for RN, if NOS)	Survival (only for RN, if NOS)	AE (for all Patients, including other diagnoses than RN, if NOS)	Comments	Lessons
Hong et al,[41] 2020	Yale University	• Case report • LITT for RN following SRS for AVM	2/2	—	—	—	AVM obliteration was confirmed before the procedure	In both cases, LITT provided a rapid resolution/stabilization of symptoms with decrease in edema
Kim et al,[25] 2020	14 centers from the LAANTERN registry[a]	• Multicenter prospective registry • LITT for intracranial tumors (including RN)	231 (223 patients)/34	—	• 1 mo: 94.1% • 3 mo: 91.1% • 6 mo: 87.8% • 12 mo: 71.1% • 24 mo: 71.1%	• 10.7% with AE • 1.8% with serious AE	—	There was no difference in the estimated OS between recurrent metastases and RN
Hong et al,[32] 2019	Yale University	• Single-center retrospective • LITT vs tumor resection for recurrent tumor after radiosurgery (recurrent metastases or RN)	34/18	• 6 mo: 87.8% without progression • 12 mo: 87.8% • 18 mo: 87.8% • 24 mo: 73.2%	• 6 mo: 94.4% • 12 mo: 73.8%–18 mo 73.8% • 24 mo: 63.2%	• Motor weakness (n = 3) • Hyperglycemia (n = 2) • Thrombocytopenia (n = 1) • Deep venous thrombosis (n = 1) • Dysphasia (n = 1) • Visual disturbance (n = 2) • Seizure (n = 2)	—	LITT showed a local control and capacity to wean off steroids similar as craniotomy and tumor resection for recurrent irradiated metastases and RN, but tumor resection was more effective to reduce neurological symptoms
Swartz et al,[42] 2019	University of Michigan Health System	• Single-center retrospective • LITT for intracranial tumors	13 (12 patients)/7	—	—	• Focal motor weakness (n = 4)	—	LITT was well tolerated and was effective in treating recurrent metastases/RN and to enable discontinuation of steroids

Study	Institution	Study design	No. lesions/patients	PFS/Survival	OS	Complications	Steroid/RN data	Key findings
Hernandez et al,[16] 2019	Rutgers University	• Single-center retrospective • LITT for recurrent metastases or RN	74 (59 patients)	44.6 wk: 83.1%	—	• New or increased motor weakness (n = 9)	No separate data for RN	• LITT should be proposed before onset of symptoms, as patients on steroids preoperative are more likely to require steroids indefinitely, as well as to experience postoperative AEs • LITT showed a significant effect on the ability to wean off steroids
Rammo et al,[43] 2018	Henry Ford Hospital	• Single-center retrospective • Safety of LITT for RN	11 (10 patients)/11	—	• 6 mo: 77.8% • 12 mo: 64.8%	• Transient new neurological deficits (n = 3) • Worsening of seizures (n = 1) • Myocardial infarction (n = 1) • Pulmonary embolus after 1 mo (n = 1)	—	• LITT was relatively safe • Significant increase in ablation volume up to 1–2 mo, then decrease to less than original volume by 6 mo (69%)
Chaunzwa et al,[35] 2018	• Yale University • Cleveland Clinic • Washington University St Louis • Wake Forest Medical Center	• Multicenter retrospective • LITT for recurrent metastases or RN	30/19	Median PFS 6 mo	• 6 mo: 52.3% • 12 mo: 26.1% • 18 mo: 21.8% • 30 mo: 16.3%	• Intraoperative hemorrhage with no need for evacuation (n = 4) • 23% of neurological/medical complication • 20% of new neurological deficits	• No separate data for RN • 73.3% of patients stopped steroids at a median time of 4.5 wk • 48% saw improvement of their preoperative symptoms	• LITT for recurrent metastases/RN may be best suited for patients with large lesions, high functional status, and stable systemic disease • Good cell death coverage (ablation volume) improves outcome
Ahluwalia et al,[24] 2018	• Cleveland Clinic • Wake Forest University	• Multicenter prospective • LITT for recurrent metastases or RN	42/19	• 12 wk: 100% without progression • 12–26 wk (last fu): 91%	• 12 wk: 100% • 26 wk: 82.1%	• Complete hemiparesis (n = 1) • Incomplete hemiparesis with hemineglect (n = 1)	—	LITT was shown prospectively to stabilize functional status, preserve quality

(continued on next page)

Table 1
(continued)

Authors	Center	Study Type and Purpose	n LITT/n LITT for RN	Progression (only for RN, if NOS)	Survival (only for RN, if NOS)	AE (for all Patients, including other diagnoses than RN, if NOS)	Comments	Lessons
	• University of Kansas • Washington University • Thomas Jefferson University and Yale University					• Headache (n = 1) • The aforementioned AEs occurred following LITT for RN		of life and cognition, and reduce the need of steroids for recurrent metastases and RN
Borghei-Razavi et al,[27] 2018	Cleveland Clinic	• Single-center retrospective case series • LITT for posterior fossa tumors	8/2	Patient 1: • Increase in lesion volume of 20% 1 day postoperative • Decrease of 30% 6 mo postoperative Patient 2: • Increase of 164% • No other fu	—	• Hydrocephalus (n=1) • Wound infection (n = 1) • Abducens nerve palsy (n = 1) • Only one AE in patients treated for RN (hydrocephalus)	—	• LITT was safe for posterior fossa lesions
Song & Colaco,[44] 2018	The Christie NHS Foundation Trust	• Case report • LITT for RN	2 (1 patient)/1	• Both lesions stable 30 mo after diagnosis of metastases (15 mo and 2 mo after LITT)		—	—	• LITT was safe and effective for local control of RN
Beechar et al,[15] 2018	Baylor College of Medicine	• Single-center retrospective • Volumetric change of recurrent metastases or RN treated with LITT	50 (36 patients)/ 50 (recurrent metastases or RN)	• Median PFS 295 days (n = 3, range 269–538 days)	• Median OS not reached	• Neurological deficits (n = 16)	• 14 lesions with sustained increased volume following LITT • No separate data for RN	• LITT resulted in an immediate increase in edema and lesion volume, followed by a gradual decrease and symptom improvement • Smaller tumors are associated with a better response

Study	Institution	Details	N	PFS	Mean survival	Complications	Notes	Conclusion
Kamath et al,[45] 2017	Washington University School of Medicine	• Single-center retrospective • LITT for intracerebral lesions	133 (120 patients)/5 RN	—	—	• Edema requiring treatment (n = 3) • Hydrocephalus (n = 3) • Meningitis (n = 1) • Seizure (n = 5) • Hemorrhage (n = 1) • Hyponatremia (n = 3) • Mild confusion (n =1)	No separate results for RN	LITT was safe and effective in a variety of intracranial lesions
Habboub et al,[31] 2017	Cleveland Clinic	• Case report • Patient with RN who underwent LITT followed by minimal invasive tumor debulking	1/1	—	—	—	Steroids weaning over 2 wk	LITT may be used in combination with tumor debulking in patients with large RN
Torcuator et al,[14] 2016	Brigham and Women's Hospital	• Case report • LITT for recurrent metastases or RN	2/unknown	—	—	• Transient word-finding difficulty (n = 1) • Transient right leg weakness (n = 1) • Both due to increased edema around the lesion	• Results of biopsy unknown • Patient 1: initial increase in edema with word-finding difficulty, 22 wk fu with decreased lesion size and edema, neurological improvement and cessation of steroids • Patient 2: slight right leg weakness at 8 wk with increase in edema and lesion size	LITT was associated with an initial increase in lesion size responding to low-dose steroids
Smith et al,[21] 2016	Barrow neurological institute	• Single-center retrospective • LITT for RN	25/25	PFS: • 11.4 mo for metastases • 8.5 mo for grade 3 lesions (WHO) • 9.1 mo for grade 4 lesions	Mean survival: • 19.2 mo for metastases • 12.2 mo for grade 3 lesions • 13.1 mo for grade 4 lesions	• Initial increased left weakness (n = 2) • Increased foot weakness (n = 1) • Steroid-induced hyperglycemia (n = 1) • Headache (n = 1) • Fatigue (n = 1) • Seizure (n = 1)	• All biopsies showed no evidence of recurrent neoplasm • In 4 cases (glioblastoma), tumor resection was required and recurrent	• LITT caused an initial increase in tumor volume with a decrease in enhancement, followed by an eventual volume decrease in

(continued on next page)

Table 1
(continued)

Authors	Center	Study Type and Purpose	n LITT/n LITT for RN	Progression (only for RN, if NOS)	Survival (only for RN, if NOS)	AE (for all Patients, including other diagnoses than RN, if NOS)	Comments	Lessons
						• Urinary retention and constipation (n = 1) • Asymptomatic catheter track hemorrhage (n = 1)	glioblastoma was found	almost all patients • LITT combined with needle biopsy may be subject to sampling error
Wright et al,[30] 2016	Cleveland Clinic	• Single-center retrospective • LITT immediately followed by minimally invasive, transsulcal resection	10/1 (with both recurrence and RN)	• No progression after 108 days	• Alive after 108 days	• Persistent mild neurological deficits (n = 1) • Transient mild neurological deficits (n = 1)		LITT may be used in combination with minimal invasive resection for difficult-to-access brain tumors
Patel et al,[13] 2016	Robert Wood Johnson University Hospital	• Single-center retrospective • LITT for various indications (including RN)	133 (102 patients)/37 (recurrent metastases or RN)	—	—	• Neurological deficits (n = 7) • Hemorrhage (n = 1) • Edema (n = 1) • Infection (n = 1) • Thermal injury (n = 1) • The aforementioned AEs occurred following LITT for recurrent metastases/RN	—	LITT resulted in few AEs that were mostly transient
Chan et al,[26] 2016	Medical College of Wisconsin	• Case report • Technical note about robot-assisted LITT for posterior fossa RN	1/1	2 mo: complete resolution of the lesion	—	—	Robot assistance was used because the trajectory was too low for arc-based stereotaxy	LITT using robot assistance in the posterior fossa was effective in inducing resolution of the lesion and improvement of symptoms

Study	Institution	Study design	n	PFS	OS	AE	PRO	Conclusions
Fabiano and Alberico[12] 2014	University at Buffalo	• Case report • LITT for recurrent metastasis or RN	1/1	—	—	—	• Preoperative steroids with adverse effects (hyperglycemia, weight gain, muscle weakness) • Postoperative steroid weaning over 2 wk	• LITT may help to reduce steroid need in patients with recurrent metastasis/RN
Rao et al,[11] 2014	Robert Wood Johnson University Hospital	• Single-center retrospective • LITT for recurrent metastases or RN	15 (14 patients)/15 (recurrent metastases or RN)	• 24 wk: 75.8% without progression • Median PFS of 37 wk	• 57% of survival median fu of 39 wk	• Asymptomatic hemorrhage (n = 1) • New left-sided weakness requiring steroids for 2 wk (n = 1)	• No distinction between recurrent metastases/RN • 5 death of extracranial disease progression • 1 death of neurological progression elsewhere	• LITT was effective and safe for patients with recurrent metastases/RN
Torres-Reveron et al,[20] 2013	Yale University	• Singe-center retrospective • LITT for recurrent metastases/RN	6/6	• 1 patient showed tumor growth after 3 mo and the tumor was resected	—	—	• 3 patients showed signs of tumor progression/recurrence on imaging, but all biopsies showed no tumor recurrence • All patients weaned of steroids by 2 mo postoperative • 1 patient died of progression of systemic disease within 1 mo	• There was a discrepancy between results of imaging and histopathology
Rahmathulla et al,[10] 2012	Cleveland Clinic	• Case report • LITT for RN	1	—	—	• Word-finding difficulty and conduction dysphasia in the immediate postoperative period	• 7 wk fu: successfully weaned off steroids, near-total resolution for neurological symptoms	• LITT was well tolerated and provided good edema and symptoms control

Abbreviations: AE, adverse events; AVM, arteriovenous malformation; fu, follow-up; IQR, interquartile range; LITT, laser interstitial thermal therapy; mo, months; NOS, not otherwise specified; OS, overall survival; PFS, progression-free survival; PRO, patient-reported outcome; RN, radiation necrosis; wk, weeks.

[a] Washington University, Wake Forest University School of Medicine, University of Texas MDA cancer center, University of California San Diego, University of Minnesota, Duke University Medical Center, Yale University, Barrow Neurological Institute, University of Louisville, Thomas Jefferson University, University Hospitals Cleveland Medical Center, SUNY upstate medical university, Florida Hospital Advent Health, Icahn School of Medicine at Mount Sinai.

tumors (mostly metastases), but the pathologies were usually not discriminated and often reported as a single entity, which hindered a better understanding of both entities.[7] Most of these studies reported promising results, as LITT for RN/recurrent metastases was considered safe, provided a good local control, enabled reduction/discontinuation of steroids, and/or reduced neurological symptoms.[11–19] Highlighting the difficulty to diagnose RN adequately, Torres-Reveron and colleagues[20] published a case series of 6 patients in which no biopsy showed evidence of tumor recurrence, whereas imaging was consistent with tumor recurrence/progression. Most interestingly, one lesion that had started regrowing after an initial decrease in size was eventually resected and diagnosed as tumor recurrence. The distinction between RN and tumor recurrence was even deliberately omitted by some investigators, as they considered that the treatment strategy could be effective regardless of the diagnosis.[11,16]

However, more recent studies tend to differentiate both pathologies, and there are multiple reports of the postoperative course of LITT for RN specifically. For example, Smith and colleagues[21] reported the results of 25 patients treated with LITT for RN following treatment of primary brain tumors and metastases. They observed a progression-free survival of 11.4 months for RN following metastases, 8.5 months for grade 3 lesions, and 9.1 months for grade 4 lesions. The corresponding mean survival was 19.2, 12.2, and 13.1 months. They reported 9 AEs (36%). In 4 cases (16%, all grade 4 lesions), tumor resection was needed after recurrence, which further highlights that stereotactic biopsy may be subject to sampling error. Later, in a subgroup of 20 patients who received LITT for RN, Shah and colleagues[22] reported a median overall survival of 16.4 months, with only 25% of the patients showing a recurrence of the lesion during the study period. They found no AE in the RN subgroup but reported a surprisingly low rate of AEs as compared with the rest of the literature (4,4%). Lanier and colleagues[23] also reported the results of LITT for 30 patients with RN, with 95.7% of patients showing no progression after 3 months, 90.9% after 6 months, and 90.9% after 9 months. The median survival was 2.1 years, with 18 patients (60%) still alive at the end of the study. They observed only 2 recurrences within 4 months, and 2 AEs (6.7%), with stable well-being and functionality measures postoperatively.

The first prospective study on this subject was published by Ahluwalia and colleagues[24] in 2018 who evaluated the outcome of LITT for recurrent metastases and RN following radiotherapy. They found a significant difference in the rate of absence of progression at 12 weeks (100% for RN vs 54% for recurrent metastases, $P < .001$), as well as survival at 12 weeks (100% for RN and 71% for recurrent metastases, $P = .02$). The difference in survival between both groups at 26 weeks was not statistically significant (82.1% for RN, 64.5% for recurrent metastases, $P = .09$). There were 3 AEs in the RN group (15.8%). Later, Kim and colleagues[25] published results from a multicenter prospective registry from which 34 patients had RN, with a survival of 94.1% after 1 month, 91.1% after 3 months, 87,8% after 6 months, and 71.1% after 24 months.

Further Applications and Comparison with Other Therapeutic Modalities

LITT for RN was shown to be safe and effective also in the posterior fossa,[26–29] and some investigators have reported good results for LITT combined with tumor debulking or resection.[30,31] Others have compared the safety and efficacy of LITT with alternative therapeutic modalities in retrospective studies. For example, Hong and colleagues[32] found that tumor resection was more effective to reduce neurological symptoms than LITT, but both interventions resulted in a comparable local control, ability to wean from steroids, and safety profile. They concluded that LITT should be considered in asymptomatic patients (or when neurological improvement is not the main purpose of the treatment) with difficult to access lesions, whereas craniotomy should be reserved for patients showing neurological symptoms and easily accessible lesions. Sujijantarat and colleagues[33] compared the outcome of LITT and bevacizumab and found that patients treated with LITT lived longer (median overall survival 24.8 months vs 15.2 months, $P = .003$), and although LITT usually resulted in an initial increase in lesional volume, the trend reversed after 1 year, as patients treated with LITT showed a median volume decrease of 64.7%, whereas those treated with bevacizumab showed a lesion volume increase of greater than 100% ($P = .01$). Finally, Sankey and colleagues[34] compared the effect of LITT and medical treatment (steroids) for biopsy-proven RN after stereotactic radiosurgery for brain metastases. They found that patients who underwent LITT were weaned from steroids more frequently (84% vs 53%, $P = .017$) and less patients developed radiographic progression in the LITT group (27% vs 5%, $P = .031$). They reported no major AEs, with a similar rate of seizure following LITT or biopsy alone.

Ablation Volume

Multiple studies have shown that good cell coverage is critical.[22,28,29,35] Chaunzwa and colleagues[35] reported a higher functional status for patients with recurrent metastases/RN and LITT volume of greater than 90% of lesion volume. Luther and colleagues[28,29] found that larger ablation volumes—most importantly supralesional ablation volumes—were more effective at reducing perilesional edema, improving functional status, and extending progression-free survival, while remaining safe even in the posterior fossa.

Volumetric Changes Following Laser Interstitial Thermal Therapy

Studies have shown that although some patients showed a rapid decrease in lesion size/edema, many were subject to an increase in size during the short-/medium-term period, with a subsequent decrease. Smith and colleagues[21] found that 2 months after LITT for RN, 74% of patients had an increase in lesion volume (mean relative increase 175%) and 26% a decrease (mean relative decrease of 38.7%). After 6 months, the trend was also for lesions to grow (66% with mean relative increase of 231.9%, 33% with a mean relative decrease of 26.2%). However, this trend was reversed after 12 months (44% with relative increase of 192%, 56% with relative decrease of 30.7%) and more dramatically after 24 months (17% with relative increase of 136.9%, 83% with a relative decrease of 49.1%). Beechar and colleagues[15] conducted a retrospective study to characterize volumetric changes following LITT for RN and recurrent metastases. Unfortunately, they did not provide separate results for patients with RN. They found an immediate increase in lesion size on T1 postcontrast imaging, with an eventual reduction in size after 6 months. FLAIR signal suggested perilesional edema was decreased after LITT in most of the patients, and this reduction was statistically significant after 6 months. Smaller tumors were associated with a better radiographic response.

Meta-Analyses

A recent meta-analysis comparing LITT with bevacizumab found that both treatments were equally effective in posttreatment symptomatic improvement, successful steroid taper, rate of recurrence, complete response, and progression.[36] Rates of partial response were higher for bevacizumab (79.6% vs 29.5%, $P = .001$) and of stable disease for LITT (6.6% vs 49.2%, $P = .002$). In addition, although there was no difference in the overall survival rates until 12 months, survival was significantly better at 18 months for LITT as compared with bevacizumab (46.4% vs 25%, $P = .038$).

A meta-analysis published in 2021 evaluated the effect of LITT for tumor recurrence and/or RN following stereotactic radiosurgery for brain metastases.[37] It reported a local control rate of 87.4% after 6 months (for the RN subgroup) and 76.3% after 12 months. These results were superior for RN compared with recurrent metastases (67.9% at 6 months, $P = .009$, 59.9% at 12 months, $P = .041$). However, overall survival was statistically not significantly different from the results for recurrent metastases (83.1% vs 69.2% at 6 months, $P = .104$, 66.8% vs 66.5% at 12 months, $P = .978$).

Current Studies

The authors found one registered recruiting study on this subject on clinicaltrials.gov. This randomized open-label study entitled "REMASTer: Recurrent Brain Metastases After SRS Trial" aims to compare LITT with steroids versus steroids alone for RN, as well as LITT alone versus LITT with hypofractionated radiotherapy for recurrent metastases. The study started in May 2022 and is expected to be completed by July 2026.

DISCUSSION
Brief Summary of the Results

Since the first report of LITT in a patient with RN, multiple studies have evaluated the procedure in infra- and supratentorial lesions of various origins. Its safety and effectiveness have been demonstrated (mostly retrospectively) for RN following radiotherapy for metastases, gliomas, and even arteriovenous malformations (see **Table 1**). Recent retrospective studies have shown that LITT is more successful than medical treatment at reducing steroid need, in slowing down progression, and increasing survival. In addition, a meta-analysis reported a superior overall survival at 18 months for LITT as compared with bevacizumab.[33,34,36]

Surgical Treatment of Radionecrosis

Although LITT is well tolerated in most patients, some patients may show a transient deterioration of neurological symptoms due to an initial increase in lesion size and surrounding edema. **Figs. 1** and **2** show the typical preoperative and postoperative course of LITT for RN with an initial increase of edema/lesion size with eventual shrinkage. Fortunately, this can very often be managed with short-term steroids, and in the medium-/long-term postoperative period, lesions and edema

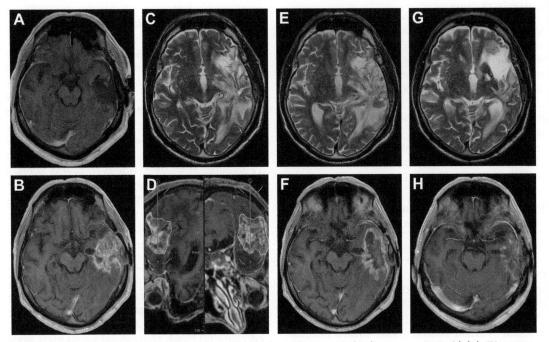

Fig. 1. Preoperative and postoperative course of LITT for radionecrosis (melanoma metastasis) (*A*). T1 postcontrast imaging after tumor resection showing no tumor remnant (*B*). T1 postcontrast imaging showing suspicion of radionecrosis (*C*). Increased T2-FLAIR signal around the lesion (edema) (*D*). Inline view of the planned LITT trajectory (*E*). Slight change of T2-FLAIR signal 1 month after LITT (*F*). T1 postcontrast imaging 1 month after LITT showing decrease of size of the lesion (*G*). Marked decrease of T2-FLAIR signal 3 months after LITT (the signal hyperintensity anterior of the lesion corresponds to cerebrospinal fluid in an old parenchymal defect and not to edema) (*H*). T1 postcontrast imaging 3 months after LITT showing significant shrinkage of the lesion.

tend to shrink, which has a net positive effect on steroid consumption.[14,16,24,35] However, this may be an important limitation in patients who present with acute neurological deficits, as rapid reduction of mass effect is of major importance and any increase in lesion volume may have dramatic consequences. In such cases, craniotomy with mass reduction may be superior to LITT.[32] As an alternative and potential future solution to this problem, there are some reports of LITT followed by minimal invasive resection.[30,31]

Indication for Laser Interstitial Thermal Therapy

RN is still not well understood, and its diagnosis and management is not well established. Therefore, arguments favoring LITT include the need for a biopsy, localization of the lesion well suited for LITT (and/or unfavorable for open resection), and resistance to steroids or taper failure.[35] Single (few) lesions and good systemic control may also be seen as essential parameters.[16,24,35] Neurological status is an important factor but there is no consensus as yet on its interpretation. Although progressing symptoms were seen as a prerequisite to use LITT by some investigators, others

advocated the use of LITT in asymptomatic patients with growing lesions, as it has been shown to be more useful when used before neurological decline/steroid dependence.[24,35,38] Because of the complexity and relativity of some of these aspects, the authors firmly believe that the decision to use LITT in such patients should be discussed in multidisciplinary tumor conferences.

Outlook and Limitations

As highlighted by multiple reports on the discrepancy between imaging and biopsy results and even discrepant biopsy results from the same lesion, diagnosing RN remains a significant challenge. Tumor recurrence and radionecrosis may be present in a single lesion, which further complicates diagnosis. Furthermore, multiple reports in the neurosurgical literature do not distinguish between the 2 entities (see **Table 1**). However, this distinction is critical, as clinical outcomes may be very different for both pathologies, and LITT has been shown to be more successful in RN than in tumor recurrence. This indiscriminate reporting is thought to introduce significant heterogeneity in the literature.[37] As an additional limitation, most reports are retrospective and

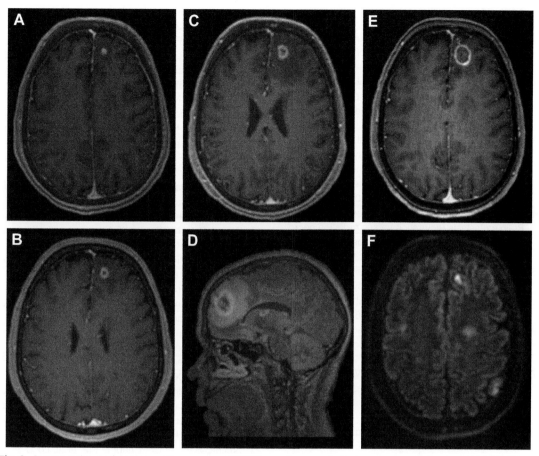

Fig. 2. Preoperative and postoperative course of LITT for radionecrosis (pulmonary carcinoma metastasis). (*A*). T1 postcontrast imaging showing the metastasis before radiation (*B*). T1 postcontrast imaging showing suspicion of radionecrosis (2 months before LITT) (*C*). T1 postcontrast imaging showing progression of the lesion (immediately before LITT) (*D*). Increased T2-FLAIR signal around the lesion (edema) during LITT (*E*). T1 postcontrast imaging showing the ablated lesion (intended to be larger than the contrast enhancing lesion) with decreased edema 1 month following LITT (*F*). Marked decrease of tumor size and of T2-FLAIR signal 3 months following LITT.

constitute small case series originating from very few institutions as shown in **Table 1**. These are severe drawbacks for evidence-based decision-making, and all efforts should be made to enroll patients in prospective registries/trials and provide as much detail about the underlying pathology as possible.

SUMMARY

In well-selected patient subgroups with lesions suspicious for RN, LITT may constitute an effective and safe treatment option and help hinder progression, lengthen survival, reduce neurological symptoms, and allow for successful steroid taper. Yet, the scientific literature on this subject is still scarce, mostly retrospective, and limited by a strong discrepancy in the classification of lesions and reported outcome measures. LITT for RN has become an additional tool for neurosurgeons to benefit patient

prognosis and quality of life, which randomized controlled studies will need to prove.

DISCLOSURE

The authors report no competing interests.

CLINICS CARE POINTS

- LITT helps to wean off steroids in RN
- RN is difficult to differentiate from tumor recurrence/progress
- LITT often results in initial increase in edema
- Large ablation volumes are recommended
- For RN, LITT may improve survival more effectively than medical therapy

REFERENCES

1. Brenner AW, Patel AJ. Review of current principles of the diagnosis and management of brain metastases. Front Oncol 2022;12:857622.
2. Ali FS, Arevalo O, Zorofchian S, et al. Cerebral radiation necrosis: incidence, pathogenesis, diagnostic challenges, and future opportunities. Curr Oncol Rep 2019;21(8):66.
3. Bernhardt D, König L, Grosu A, et al. DEGRO practical guideline for central nervous system radiation necrosis part 1: classification and a multistep approach for diagnosis. Strahlenther Onkol 2022. https://doi.org/10.1007/s00066-022-01994-3.
4. Lee D, Riestenberg RA, Haskell-Mendoza A, et al. Brain metastasis recurrence versus radiation necrosis: evaluation and treatment. Neurosurg Clin N Am 2020;31(4):575–87.
5. Bernhardt D, König L, Grosu AL, et al. DEGRO practical guideline for central nervous system radiation necrosis part 2: treatment. Strahlenther Onkol 2022. https://doi.org/10.1007/s00066-022-01973-8.
6. Yang X, Ren H, Fu J. Treatment of radiation-induced brain necrosis. Oxid Med Cel Longev 2021;2021:4793517.
7. Bastos DCA, Weinberg J, Kumar VA, et al. Laser interstitial thermal therapy in the treatment of brain metastases and radiation necrosis. Cancer Lett 2020;489:9–18.
8. Carpentier A, McNichols RJ, Stafford RJ, et al. Real-time magnetic resonance-guided laser thermal therapy for focal metastatic brain tumors. Neurosurgery 2008;63(1 Suppl 1):ONS21–8.
9. Carpentier A, McNichols RJ, Stafford RJ, et al. Laser thermal therapy: real-time MRI-guided and computer-controlled procedures for metastatic brain tumors. Lasers Surg Med 2011;43(10):943–50.
10. Rahmathulla G, Recinos PF, Valerio JE, et al. Laser interstitial thermal therapy for focal cerebral radiation necrosis: a case report and literature review. Stereotact Funct Neurosurg 2012;90(3):192–200.
11. Rao MS, Hargreaves EL, Khan AJ, et al. Magnetic resonance-guided laser ablation improves local control for postradiosurgery recurrence and/or radiation necrosis. Neurosurgery 2014;74(6):658–67.
12. Fabiano AJ, Alberico RA. Laser-interstitial thermal therapy for refractory cerebral edema from post-radiosurgery metastasis. World Neurosurg 2014;81(3–4):652.e1–4.
13. Patel P, Patel NV, Danish SF. Intracranial MR-guided laser-induced thermal therapy: single-center experience with the Visualase thermal therapy system. J Neurosurg 2016;125(4):853–60.
14. Torcuator RG, Hulou MM, Chavakula V, et al. Intraoperative real-time MRI-guided stereotactic biopsy followed by laser thermal ablation for progressive brain metastases after radiosurgery. J Clin Neurosci 2016;24:68–73.
15. Beechar VB, Prabhu SS, Bastos D, et al. Volumetric response of progressing post-SRS lesions treated with laser interstitial thermal therapy. J Neurooncol 2018;137(1):57–65.
16. Hernandez RN, Carminucci A, Patel P, et al. Magnetic resonance-guided laser-induced thermal therapy for the treatment of progressive enhancing inflammatory reactions following stereotactic radiosurgery, or PEIRs, for metastatic brain disease. Neurosurgery 2019;85(1):84–90.
17. Ginalis EE, Danish SF. Magnetic resonance-guided laser interstitial thermal therapy for brain tumors in geriatric patients. Neurosurg Focus 2020;49(4):E12.
18. Kaye J, Patel NV, Danish SF. Laser interstitial thermal therapy for in-field recurrence of brain metastasis after stereotactic radiosurgery: does treatment with LITT prevent a neurologic death? Clin Exp Metastasis 2020;37(3):435–44.
19. Riviere-Cazaux C, Bhandarkar AR, Rahman M, et al. Outcomes and principles of patient selection for laser interstitial thermal therapy for metastatic brain tumor management: a multisite institutional case series. World Neurosurg 2022. https://doi.org/10.1016/j.wneu.2022.06.095.
20. Torres-Reveron J, Tomasiewicz HC, Shetty A, et al. Stereotactic laser induced thermotherapy (LITT): a novel treatment for brain lesions regrowing after radiosurgery. J Neurooncol 2013;113(3):495–503.
21. Smith CJ, Myers CS, Chapple KM, et al. Long-term follow-up of 25 cases of biopsy-proven radiation necrosis or post-radiation treatment effect treated with magnetic resonance-guided laser interstitial thermal therapy. Neurosurgery 2016;79(Suppl 1):S59–72.
22. Shah AH, Semonche A, Eichberg DG, et al. The role of laser interstitial thermal therapy in surgical neuro-oncology: series of 100 consecutive patients. Neurosurgery 2020;87(2):266–75.
23. Lanier CM, Lecompte M, Glenn C, et al. A single-institution retrospective study of patients treated with laser-interstitial thermal therapy for radiation necrosis of the brain. Cureus. 2021;13(11):e19967.
24. Ahluwalia M, Barnett GH, Deng D, et al. Laser ablation after stereotactic radiosurgery: a multicenter prospective study in patients with metastatic brain tumors and radiation necrosis. J Neurosurg 2018;130(3):804–11.
25. Kim AH, Tatter S, Rao G, et al. Laser ablation of abnormal neurological tissue using robotic neuroblate system (laantern): 12-month outcomes and quality of life after brain tumor ablation. Neurosurgery 2020;87(3):E338–46.
26. Chan AY, Tran DK, Gill AS, et al. Stereotactic robot-assisted MRI-guided laser thermal ablation of radiation necrosis in the posterior cranial fossa: technical note. Neurosurg Focus 2016;41(4):E5.

27. Borghei-Razavi H, Koech H, Sharma M, et al. Laser interstitial thermal therapy for posterior fossa lesions: an initial experience. World Neurosurg 2018; 117:e146–53.

28. Luther E, Lu VM, Morell AA, et al. Supralesional ablation volumes are feasible in the posterior fossa and may provide enhanced symptomatic relief. Oper Neurosurg (Hagerstown) 2021;21(6):418–25.

29. Luther E, McCarthy D, Shah A, et al. Radical laser interstitial thermal therapy ablation volumes increase progression-free survival in biopsy-proven radiation necrosis. World Neurosurg 2020;136:e646–59.

30. Wright J, Chugh J, Wright CH, et al. Laser interstitial thermal therapy followed by minimal-access transsulcal resection for the treatment of large and difficult to access brain tumors. Neurosurg Focus 2016;41(4):E14.

31. Habboub G, Sharma M, Barnett GH, et al. A novel combination of two minimally invasive surgical techniques in the management of refractory radiation necrosis: technical note. J Clin Neurosci 2017;35: 117–21.

32. Hong CS, Deng D, Vera A, et al. Laser-interstitial thermal therapy compared to craniotomy for treatment of radiation necrosis or recurrent tumor in brain metastases failing radiosurgery. J Neurooncol 2019; 142(2):309–17.

33. Sujijantarat N, Hong CS, Owusu KA, et al. Laser interstitial thermal therapy (LITT) vs. bevacizumab for radiation necrosis in previously irradiated brain metastases. J Neurooncol 2020;148(3):641–9.

34. Sankey EW, Grabowski MM, Srinivasan ES, et al. Time to steroid independence after laser interstitial thermal therapy vs medical management for treatment of biopsy-proven radiation necrosis secondary to stereotactic radiosurgery for brain metastasis. Neurosurgery 2022;90(6):684–90.

35. Chaunzwa TL, Deng D, Leuthardt EC, et al. Laser thermal ablation for metastases failing radiosurgery: a multicentered retrospective study. Neurosurgery 2018;82(1):56–63.

36. Palmisciano P, Haider AS, Nwagwu CD, et al. Bevacizumab vs laser interstitial thermal therapy in cerebral radiation necrosis from brain metastases: a systematic review and meta-analysis. J Neurooncol 2021;154(1):13–23.

37. Chen C, Guo Y, Chen Y, et al. The efficacy of laser interstitial thermal therapy for brain metastases with in-field recurrence following SRS: systemic review and meta-analysis. Int J Hyperthermia 2021; 38(1):273–81.

38. Hong CS, Beckta JM, Kundishora AJ, et al. Laser interstitial thermal therapy for treatment of cerebral radiation necrosis. Int J Hyperthermia 2020;37(2): 68–76.

39. Bastos DCA, Rao G, Oliva ICG, et al. Predictors of local control of brain metastasis treated with laser interstitial thermal therapy. Neurosurgery 2020; 87(1):112–22.

40. Shao J, Radakovich NR, Grabowski M, et al. Lessons learned in using laser interstitial thermal therapy for treatment of brain tumors: a case series of 238 patients from a single institution. World Neurosurg 2020;139:e345–54.

41. Hong CS, Cord BJ, Kundishora AJ, et al. MRI-guided laser interstitial thermal therapy for radiation necrosis in previously irradiated brain arteriovenous malformations. Pract Radiat Oncol 2020;10(4): e298–303.

42. Swartz LK, Holste KG, Kim MM, et al. Outcomes in patients treated with laser interstitial thermal therapy for primary brain cancer and brain metastases. Oncologist 2019;24(12):e1467–70.

43. Rammo R, Asmaro K, Schultz L, et al. The safety of magnetic resonance imaging-guided laser interstitial thermal therapy for cerebral radiation necrosis. J Neurooncol 2018;138(3):609–17.

44. Song YP, Colaco RJ. Radiation necrosis - a growing problem in a case of brain metastases following whole brain radiotherapy and stereotactic radiosurgery. Cureus. 2018;10(1):e2037.

45. Kamath AA, Friedman DD, Hacker CD, et al. MRI-guided interstitial laser ablation for intracranial lesions: a large single-institution experience of 133 cases. Stereotact Funct Neurosurg 2017;95(6): 417–28.

Posterior Fossa Laser Interstitial Thermal Therapy in Children

Giuseppe Mirone, MD, Domenico Cicala, MD, Giuseppe Cinalli, MD*

KEYWORDS

- Laser interstitial thermal therapy • Tumor ablation • Posterior fossa • Brainstem • Minimally invasive
- Pediatric tumor • Magnetic resonance imaging • Cavernous malformation

KEY POINTS

- MRI-guided laser interstitial thermal therapy (MRgLITT) is an emerging technique to treat posterior fossa lesions.
- Pediatric posterior fossa MRgLITT is extremely demanding due to the anatomical complexity of the region (concentration of eloquent areas, bone anatomy, dural sinuses) and to the limitations of the technology currently available for the pediatric population.
- We report our experience and analyze the current literature on MRgLITT for the treatment of posterior fossa in children.

▶ Video content accompanies this article at http://www.neurosurgery.theclinics.com.

INTRODUCTION

Pediatric posterior fossa brain tumors can be managed using a variety of surgical procedures depending on the tumor's location and histology. The most frequent treatment of accessible brain tumors is surgical resection with an open craniotomy. The highest chance of survival or long-term tumor control typically comes from total or almost complete surgical removal in the vast majority of histological subtypes. Complication rates for surgical resection in these patients based on current evidence is approximately 26%.[1] Radiation and/or chemotherapy, which can have severe long-term damage in children, are the only treatments available for tumors that cannot be removed surgically or that are resistant to surgical intervention[2–4]

As a less invasive surgical approach, MRI-guided laser interstitial thermal treatment (MRgLITT) can be used to treat brain tumors, especially if deep-seated or in eloquent areas. Through the application of laser light administered to a target, cell death is caused by time-dependent thermal damage to intracellular proteins and DNA. When paired with the capacity to monitor and manage the ablation via MR thermal imaging, this technique offers a sharp separation between ablated and unaffected tissue, resulting in a high level of precision and control.

The early results of MRgLITT for deep brain lesions that are surgically inoperable, such as lesions in the thalamus, hypothalamus, basal ganglia, and brainstem, are encouraging.[5–9] In addition, MRgLITT may be used to treat tumors that have recurred or persisted despite previous treatment.

The few small series trying to assess the efficacy of MRgLITT in the posterior fossa have mostly involved adult patients.[1,10–13] The use of the LITT in pediatric diseases of the posterior fossa is more difficult and demanding due to the

Department of Pediatric Neurosurgery, Santobono-Pausilipon Children's Hospital, AORN, Via Mario Fiore 6 80121, Napoli, Italy
* Corresponding author.
E-mail address: giuseppe.cinalli@gmail.com

Neurosurg Clin N Am 34 (2023) 227–237
https://doi.org/10.1016/j.nec.2022.11.002
1042-3680/23/© 2022 Elsevier Inc. All rights reserved.

anatomical complexity of the region (concentration of eloquent areas, bone anatomy, dural sinuses) and to the limitations of the technology currently available for the pediatric population.

We reviewed the current available literature and presented our preliminary experience with the use of MRgLITT for the treatment of pediatric brain tumors and cavernous malformations (CM) in this complex anatomical location.

Materials and Methods

This was a retrospective single-institution review of patients with posterior fossa lesions treated by MRgLITT at Santobono-Pausilipon Children's Hospital (Naples, Italy). Data were obtained from clinical records, operative notes, and radiological files from January 2019 to August 2022. Patients were ultimately considered candidates for LITT based on the clinical judgment of a multidisciplinary board. The demographics, lesion volume, clinical history, LITT procedural data, and indications for surgery are reported in **Table 1**. Lesion volume was calculated preoperatively and postoperatively based on MRI measurements and the assumption that the tumors were ellipsoid.

Routine postoperative visits occurred at 2 weeks and then at 3 months after surgery. Postoperative MRI was performed every 3 months to evaluate tumor size and volume.

We reviewed also published articles in English with no limits on the year of publication until August 2022. The following databases were searched: Medline, PubMed, Scopus, and Cochrane to find details on the effectiveness and safety of LITT in pediatric posterior fossa lesions. The following keywords and terms were used in this study: "Laser Interstitial Thermal Therapy" OR "LITT" OR "Laser ablation" AND "brainstem" OR "cerebellum" OR "posterior fossa" OR "posterior cranial fossa" OR "pediatric" OR "pons" OR "midbrain" OR "children".

RESULTS

Clinical and surgical data are shown in **Table 1**. We identified four patients (three boys and one girl). Mean age was 8.5 years (6 to 12 years). Indications were recurrence of residual tumor in three patients operated for posterior fossa pilocytic astrocytoma in three patients and a bleeding cavernoma in one patient. All MRgLITT procedures were performed using the Visualase thermal laser system (Medtronic, Minneapolis, MN, USA). For all patients a single lesion was treated in one single robotic-assisted (Stealth Autoguide, Medtronic, Minneapolis, MN, USA) frameless MRgLITT procedure: two 10 mm fibers and two 3 mm fibers

were used depending on the size of the lesion and, in two cases, one single pullback of the fiber was performed to enhance the area of the ablation (**Table 1**). Locations were the superior cerebellar peduncle in two cases and middle cerebellar peduncle in two cases. The median preoperative volume was 2.57 cm^3 (1.36 to 4.61 cm^3). The mean postoperative volume at the last neuroradiological follow-up was 1.31 cm^3 (0.15 to 2.41 cm^3).

Mean clinical and radiological follow-up was 18.5 months (4 to 36 months). There were no deaths and one permanent complication (unilateral hearing loss). Dexamethasone was started the day before LITT at a dose of (0.5 mg/kg) and continued with a 2-week weaning plan to reduce postoperative cerebral edema.

Case Illustrations

Case no. 1

An 8-year-old boy presented with a headache and a 2-week history of diplopia and a stiff neck with a deviation of the head downwards and to the right (Video 1, **Fig. 1** A-D). History was positive for familiar cavernomatosis. A computed tomography (CT) scan revealed a subacute bleeding at the level of the right middle cerebellar peduncle and additional lesions were reported at the lateral wall of the left ventricular trigone and in the left striatum. Further characterization with MRI confirmed cavernomatosis and a rounded cavernoma with subacute bleeding in the posterior fossa. The patient was offered thermal ablation of the cerebellar cavernoma by MRgLITT. We decided to create a three-dimensional (3D)-printed model of the head for surgical simulation and planning. Laser ablation was delivered along trans-cerebellar trajectory. Treatment was completed without intraoperative complication. In the first few days after surgery patient had vertigo, dizziness, and dysmetria that after 4 weeks disappeared with a residual unilateral hearing loss. Follow-up MRI at 3 months showed a persistent T1-weighted Gd-enhancing signal consistent with successful laser ablation and subsequent controls showed a progressive reduction and disappearance of the lesion. Unilateral hearing loss did not recover at 2-year follow-up.

Case no. 2

An 11-year-old boy presented for worsening headache and vomiting (Video 2, **Fig. 1** E-H). MRI scan revealed a cerebellar tumor associated with triventricular hydrocephalus. He underwent subtotal removal of the lesion through a suboccipital approach. Histology revealed a pilocytic astrocytoma.

Follow-up MRI (at 3 and 6 months) showed a growing residual tumor at the level of the right

Table 1
Clinical and surgical data of pediatric patients treated by MRI-guided laser interstitial thermal treatment at Santobono-Pausilipon Children's Hospital

Patient No.	Gender	Age	Location	Pathology	Previous Treatments	Pre-/Post-Ablation Lesion Volume (cm³)	No. of Fibers (Type)/No. of Pullback	Laser Treatment	Follow-up (mos)	Complications
No. 1	M	8	Right middle cerebellar peduncle	Cavernous Malformation	None	1.36/0.15	1 (3 mm)/1	6.10 W for 78 s 5.00 W for 110 s *5.10 W for 116 s*	24	Unilateral hearing loss
No. 2	M	14	Right superior cerebellar peduncle	Pilocytic Astrocytoma	Suboccipital Craniotomy	2.21/1.84	1 (10 mm)/2	4.50 W for 34 s 9.15 W for 51 s 7.35 W for 75 s *4.50 W for 195 s* *8.10 W for 135 s* *4.50 W for 78 s* *8.10 W for 42 s*	32	None
No. 3	M	6	Left superior cerebellar peduncle	Pilocytic Astrocytoma	Suboccipital Craniotomy	2.11/0.87	1 (3 mm)/0	2.00 W for 77 s 5.10 W for 38 s 5.10 W for 176 s 7.00 W for 156 s	4	None
No. 4	F	10	Right middle cerebellar peduncle	Pilocytic Astrocytoma	Retrosigmoid Craniotomy	4.61/2.41	1 (10 mm)/2	3.00 W for 38 s 5.10 W for 39 s 4.50 W for 28 s 4.00 W for 128 s *2.80 W for 84 s* *2.80 W for 77 s* *4.10 W for 97 s*	14	None

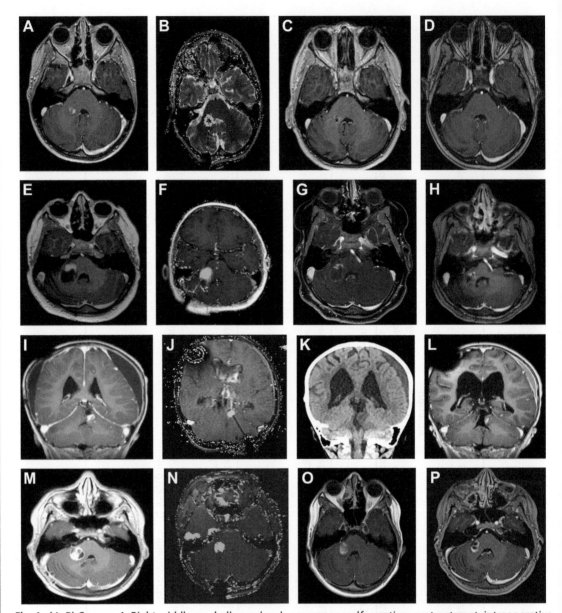

Fig. 1. (A–D) Case no. 1: Right middle cerebellar peduncle cavernous malformation: pretreatment, intraoperative ablation and follow-up MRI at 3 months and 18 months. (E–H) Case no. 2: Right superior cerebellar peduncle progression of residual pilocytic astrocytoma: pretreatment, intraoperative ablation and follow-up MRI at 3 months and 32 months. (I–L) Case no. 3: Left superior cerebellar peduncle progression of residual pilocytic astrocytoma: pretreatment, intraoperative ablation, postoperative CT scan and follow-up MRI at 3 months. (M–P) Case no. 4: Right middle cerebellar peduncle progression of residual pilocytic astrocytoma: pretreatment, intraoperative ablation and follow-up MRI at 3 months and 12 months.

superior cerebellar peduncle. MRgLITT was performed by a trans cerebellar trajectory. On day 2 postoperative patients were discharged without complications with a normal neurological examination. Follow-up MRIs at 24 months showed nearly total ablation of the tumor with no signs of regrowth.

Case no. 3

A 6-year-old boy presented for worsening balance with repeated fall (**Fig. 1** I-L, **Fig. 2** E-F, **Fig. 3**D and **Fig. 4**). Neurological examination confirmed an uncertain walking with impairment of fine motor skills. Ophthalmological evaluation revealed bilateral papilledema.

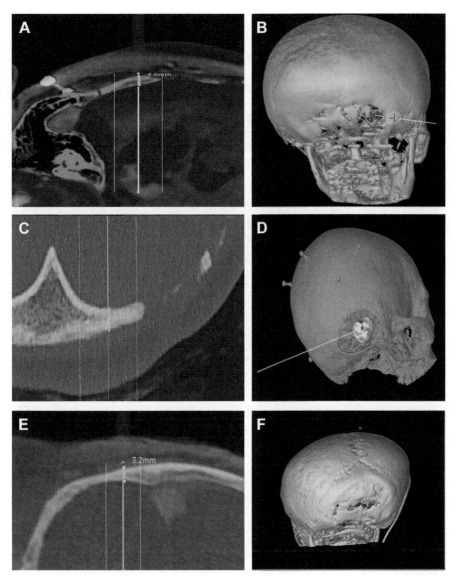

Fig. 2. Preoperative planning for Case no. 2 (*A, B*), Case no. 3 (*E, F*), and Case no. 4 (*C, D*) considering skull thickness at the entry point and previous craniotomies.

An MRI showed a voluminous posterior fossa tumor with secondary hydrocephalus. The patient underwent an endoscopic third ventriculostomy followed by microsurgical removal of the lesion by a suboccipital approach. Histology revealed a pilocytic astrocytoma.

After 2 weeks a ventriculoperitoneal shunt was implanted for persistent hydrocephalus. Follow-up MRI at 6 months showed a growing residual tumor at the level of the right superior cerebellar peduncle and upper vermis. MRgLITT was performed without complications by a transcerebellar trajectory. The patient was discharged after 2 days. Follow-up MRI after MRgLITT at

3 months showed subtotal ablation of the residual tumor with no signs of recurrence.

Case no. 4 (alvario)

A 10-year-old girl presented for 1-month history of headache, dizziness, and walking difficulties (**Fig. 1** M-P, **Fig. 2** C-D). An MRI showed a mainly cystic tumor at the level of the right middle cerebellar peduncle extending to the right cerebellopontine angle (CPA) angle. She underwent subtotal microsurgical removal through a retro sigmoid approach. The residual solid component of the tumor showed progressive regrowth at 3 months follow-up MRI, she underwent MRgLITT

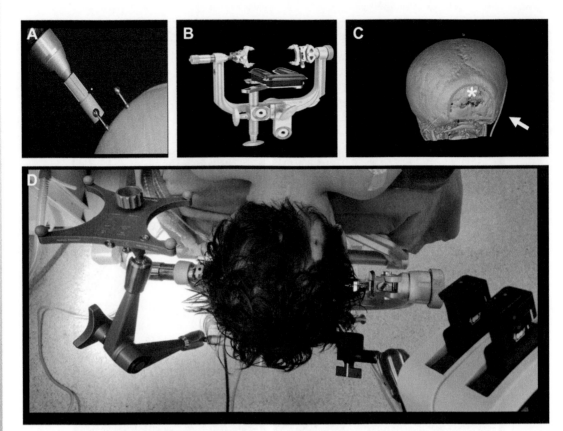

Fig. 3. Surgical key points for pediatric posterior fossa MRgLITT. (*A*) Bone fiducials (at least five) are implanted to enhance precision. (*B*) Four pediatric pins plus additional gel head ring (DORO Multi-Purpose Skull Clamp) can be used to secure the head and overcoming the minimal skull thickness in children. (*C*) Surgical planning must consider skull thickness at the entry point, previous craniotomies (*) and shunts (*white arrow*). (*D*) Intraoperative images demonstrating patient's positioning (Case no. 3) with the robotic arm (Stealth Autoguide, Medtronic, Minneapolis, MN, USA). We prefer Minimal hair removal for posterior fossa MRgLITT and a 20 to 30 mm skin incision because of occipital muscles.

through a trans-cerebellar trajectory 5 months after the first surgery. Laser ablation was completed without complication. The patient was discharged the day after surgery. Follow-up MRIs 14 months after LITT showed no sign of further recurrence.

Posterior Fossa MRI-Guided Laser Interstitial Thermal Therapy Workflow

The whole workflow of the procedure must be proven and standardized. In our first case of posterior fossa MRgLITT, we decided to create a 3D-printed patient-specific anatomical model for surgical planning. In this way, the day before surgery, we were able to simulate the surgical procedure, check the input trajectory, assess the best possible positioning for the patient, and mimic all surgical steps of a robotic-assisted MRgLITT in the posterior fossa, saving time in the operating room and allowing all the operating room personnel to experience the real workflow.[12]

Planning

Laser trajectories were simulated on the Stealth Guide planning station (Medtronic, Minneapolis, MN, USA) according to preoperative MRI. It is mandatory to obtain a very recently updated preoperative MRI, especially in children with ventriculoperitoneal shunt.

For pediatric posterior fossa MRgLITT, it is important to carefully analyze the relevant anatomy: tractography and, most recently, connectome images may be very helpful in this area.

The morphology of the lesion in relation to the size of the laser fiber and the ensuing shape of laser emission, as well as the basic MRgLITT principles and guidelines, must all be taken into consideration during trajectory design. To achieve the best results, planning of MRgLITT requires not only the accuracy of the target point, but also the accuracy of the trajectory so that it is possible to pull back the laser fiber along an axis to enhance the area of the ablation.

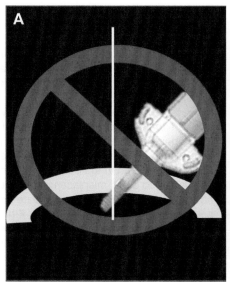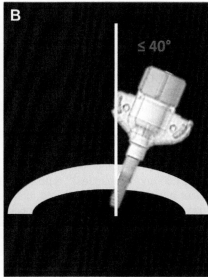

Fig. 4. Metal bone anchor should carefully anchor (*B*), without excessive angulation (*A*), to avoid misplacement because small errors at the entry point can translate into significant errors at the target level.

Excessive angulation when drilling must be avoided because it may result in skull bolt displacement or inadequate skull bolt angle when screwing the bolt: it's crucial to consider the angle and slope of the occipital bone, the craniotomy from prior surgeries, the presence of a ventriculoperitoneal (VP) shunt, and assess the thickness of the skull at the level of the entry point (**Fig. 3**C and **2** A-F). It is also essential to be aware that for trajectories where the laser fiber must pass through the ventricle or a cystic compartment, this could result in a deflection of the laser fiber and subsequent off-targeting.

The risk of thermal injury to the nearby vital tissue is further diminished if "heat sinks" such as big arteries and/or cerebrospinal fluid (CSF) spaces are close by to the target. These structures in fact dissipate the heat very rapidly due to the high speed of blood inside the arterial lumen and the pulsatile movements of CSF inside the subarachnoid spaces. This rapid dissipation certainly protects the blood vessels by reducing the risk of accidental thermal damage to their wall, and prevents thermal damage to diffuse to an adjacent gyrus due to the presence of the CSF circulating inside the sulcus. At the same time, if such a dissipating structure is included inside the ablation volume, it may be difficult to get a sufficiently homogeneous rise in target temperature inside the target due to "heat sinks," thus creating irregular ablation shapes not perfectly corresponding to the planned ablation volume.

If there is more than 1 mm between the ablation zone and the surrounding tissues, it is typically safe since the temperature at the ablation zone's edge drops off quickly.

Positioning

All procedures were performed after general anesthesia was induced. Prophylactic antibiotic was started. Our protocol included the administration of intravenous dexamethasone (0.5 mg/kg) from the day before surgery.

First, with the child in the supine position, six bone fiducials (**Fig. 3**A) are fixed and a CT scan is acquired and co-registered with the preoperative recent MRI. CT/MRI fusion may minimize effects of distortion. In our experience, for pediatric posterior fossa frameless MRgLITT, bone fiducial-based registration (with at least five fiducials) offers a higher level of accuracy and offers the possibility to keep in the surgical field some of the fiducials (usually the retro mastoid or occipital fiducials) to check the accuracy intraoperatively. It is also important to spread out the fiducials asymmetrically throughout the patient's head (error increases as the configuration of the fiducials gets narrower or symmetrical), avoiding a distorted scalp.

Highly precise stereotactic fiber insertion is necessary to operate the MRgLITT system. Frame-based or frameless neuronavigation techniques can be used. Both methods, however, entail rigidly immobilizing the head with cranial pin fixation, necessitating enough skull thickness to securely fasten the pins: as a result, only individuals aged 2 years or older are described in most pediatric cases.[14] On the contrary, children should not have their pins tightened excessively because this can lead to intracranial damage due to the penetration of the skull's inner table.

In our experience, each patient was then positioned prone with the head well fixed (DORO Multi-Purpose Skull Clamp): for young children we use four pediatric pins plus additional gel head ring to secure the head (**Fig. 3**B) and overcome the minimal skull thickness, as similarly proposed by Gupta and colleagues[15] and Lee and colleagues.[16,17]

To overcome the challenging skull fixation in young children, Lee and colleagues[16] reported a successful laser ablation in a 4-month-old infant with tuberous sclerosis complex (TSC) presenting with refractory focal seizures using a combination of AxIEM electromagnetic navigation, the Navigus biopsy platform, and the Visualase system.

At this step, the bone fiducials are manually registered (Stealth S7 , Medtronic, Minneapolis, MN, USA): acceptable navigation accuracy for posterior fossa is $\leq$ 1 mm. Persistent decrease of accuracy during surgery can be observed that is usually related to the length of surgery, draping, or drilling.

In all posterior fossa MRgLITT cases, we used a robotic guidance platform (Stealth Autoguide , Medtronic, Minneapolis, MN, USA) to enhance accuracy in the positioning of the laser fiber: between registration and surgery, the skull clamp, the small passive cranial frame, and the robotic arm need to be tightly fastened (**Fig. 3**D).

When using the Stealth Autoguide robotic arm, it's better to simulate all the possible alignments of the robot at the entry point to avoid extreme positioning of the robotic arm because the intrinsic weight of the robotic system can cause slight displacement of the planned trajectory during the drilling or the insertion of the bone anchor.

Surgical technique

The scalp entrance zone was sterilized: we prefer to shave a strip of hair for posterior fossa MRgLITT in children. To allow for appropriate posterior cervical muscle retraction before drilling, a bigger incision (20 mm) is made for the anchor bolt insertion than is necessary for supratentorial lesions. Furthermore, the posterior fossa's shape offers little bone for the bolt to anchor against. As a result, the bigger incision makes it simpler to enter the bolt in the skull perpendicular to the intended probe direction. The thickness of the skull is calculated at the entry point and a guided drill hole was made meticulously to create a single trajectory in the bone: this is the single most important factor for avoiding trajectory error.

Dural opening is achieved sharply and then coagulated using an endoscopic monopolar coagulator through the guide.

At this point, we used a navigated biopsy needle biopsy to make the path for the laser fiber at least until the limit of the lesion, even if we decided not to perform biopsy.

The bone anchor was then screwed and secured to the skull with a stylet in place. The metal bone anchor provides a better accuracy than plastic anchor and should be preferred and carefully anchored in the bone, without excessive angulation, to avoid misplacement because small errors at the entry point can translate into significant errors at the target level (see **Fig. 3**). Next, the laser insertion point and depth were marked with sterile tape at the top of the bone anchor and the cooling catheter was inserted through the bolt to the calculated target.

MRI

At this point, we carefully transfer the patient to the MRI suite. The top coil of MRI is placed, and we proceed with performing the MRI for thermal-guided ablation. Thorough attention was placed on avoiding any movement to the laser fiber and skull mount during the entire process.

3D T1-weighted fast spoiled gradient images are then acquired: it is obligatory to obtain an MRI scan before beginning thermal ablation to show the full length of the probe, to ensure accurate positioning in the lesion and to rule out any complications.

A T1 or T2-FLAIR image is then acquired to act as an anatomical reference image as a background on the Visualase workstation to overlay the real-time thermal images.

The thermal ablation plan was created by focusing three crossed low-temperature limits to protect the interface with the normal brain and one crossed high-temperature limit in the intended area of maximal ablation. To confirm the starting point for the laser emission and for laser software synchronization, a test dose with 25% of the laser's power was applied before administering treatment doses.

The ablation proceeded with the goal of creating a complete lesionectomy based on the predicted damage map.

Low-temperature limits were set to prevent injury to adjacent eloquent areas. If more thermal ablation zones were required, either a second local dosage to expand the ablation area was repeated, or the laser fiber was pulled back by 5 mm inside the cooling catheter. To create a final total ablation zone, initial and superimposed thermal ablation zones were saved. Postoperative FLAIR and T1-

weighted contrast-enhanced MR images were acquired. After that, the cooling catheter, laser probe, and anchor were taken out of the patient and placed in the recovery area. A single 3-0 absorbable suture was used to close each wound.

DISCUSSION
Posterior Fossa MRI-Guided Laser Interstitial Thermal Therapy for Tumors

The use of MRgLITT in the posterior fossa has been limited to a few series and mostly in adult patients.[1,9–12,18]

Borghei-Razavi and colleagues[11] presented a series of eight patients who underwent LITT for infratentorial metastases (three cases), radiation necrosis (two cases), pilocytic astrocytoma (two cases), and glioblastoma (one case) with a local control rate of 75%. Two tumors in this study showed progression at 8.5 months (glioblastoma) and 7.5 months (metastatic adenocarcinoma). They noted transient sixth cranial nerve palsy in one patient, which improved at 3-month follow-up

Traylor and colleagues[10] described 13 adult patients with radiation necrosis (five cases) and metastases (eight cases), who were managed using MRgLITT. Overall, there was recurrence in 69.2% of the subjects. They reported complications in one patient with radiation necrosis with permanent seventh and eighth cranial nerve palsy.

Recently, Ashraf and colleagues[12] performed the only retrospective review of the use of MRgLITT in the posterior fossa. They evaluated 58 patients (60 tumors) across four institutions. Mean age was 56.4 but no details about pediatric cases were given.

In their series, there were a total of 15 primary tumors and 45 secondary tumors (44 cases of infield recurrence and one untreated metastatic tumor), and 53 patients (91%) had undergone prior intervention for their tumor. The median preablation tumor volume was 2.24 cm³. 48 patients (50 tumors) were available for follow-up. An 84% (42/50) overall local control rate was achieved at 9.5 months median follow-up.

Tovar-Spinoza and colleagues[19] reported the use of MRgLITT in 12 tumors in 11 pediatric patients whose mean age was 10.3 years (range 4 to 17 years). Six patients underwent MRgLITT as a first-line treatment, five had undergone previous open surgery, and three had undergone oncological treatment that failed. All MRgLITT procedures were performed using the Visualase system.

They reported a 4-year-old boy with brainstem medulloblastoma and no metastatic disease who underwent resection, chemotherapy, and stem cell rescue. MRgLITT was proposed for a recurrent tumor in the left pons as a palliative treatment. The patient did not receive any additional chemotherapy after the procedure and the follow-up at 17 months found no recurrence.

The other three posterior fossa tumors (1 vermian, 1 cerebellar peduncle, and 1 tentorial) were all recurrent pilocytic astrocytoma. Mean target volume was 4.69 cm³ (1.94 to 10.55 cm³). In all cases, a single laser fiber was used with additional pulling of the laser fiber in two cases. No perioperative morbidities were reported. Mean follow-up was 16.3 months (12 to 32) and no recurrence or progression was reported. Two experienced post-ablation morbidity improving over time.

Few studies have described the use of MRgLITT for lesions specifically in the brainstem or cerebellar peduncles.

Patel and colleagues[9] reported a total of 12 patients had undergone MRgLITT for brainstem pathologies. The average age of the patients was 47.6 years (range 4 to 75 years). The pathologies included both primary and metastatic intracranial tumors. In their study, local control rate was 77.8%. The only pediatric patient was a 4-year-old child with a pontine ependymoma who underwent MRgLITT by a transcerebellar approach.

Although considerable variability was present in these studies, the high tumor control rates suggest that LITT in this region of the brain is feasible, enabling thermal ablation coverage of the target to facilitate long-term control. The added benefit of MRgLITT is the option for serial treatments if a patient experiences recurrence. However, large studies with longer follow-up periods are required to evaluate the efficacy of repeat ablation.

Posterior Fossa MRI-Guided Laser Interstitial Thermal Therapy for Cavernous Malformations

Microsurgical resection of intracranial CM is regarded as the standard treatment but in recent years, there have been reports of the application of MRgLITT for intracranial CMs.[20,21]

Lawrence and colleagues[22] reported thermal ablation of a pontine CM via a suboccipital burr hole passing through the middle cerebellar peduncle. Postoperatively, the patient was noted to have diplopia secondary to the abducent's palsy.

Gamboa and colleagues[23] showed that LITT therapy may serve as a useful alternative treatment modality in select patients to alter the natural history of brainstem CMs. They reported two adult cases in which MRgLITT therapy was used for the treatment of pontine CMs after recurrent hemorrhage. The authors used a frontal, transcapsular, and a suboccipital, transpeduncular approache to the brainstem. Only one patient experienced temporary worsened neurological function that authors associated with the frontal trajectory near the area of the internal capsule. Progressive radiographic involution of lesions and hemorrhage-free survival at 18 months and 12 months was reported.

In their systematic review, Yousefi and colleagues[24] identified six studies, reporting the outcome of 33 patients. In 26 patients, CM was found as the epileptogenic foci and in others, CM was the cause of headache or focal neurological deficits. In their review, three patients had CM in the brain stem region. Surgery-related complications occurred in 3 different cases: in one case a non-disabling visual field defect resulted from extended ablation in the temporal lobe,[20] in one case a malfunction related to the catheter causing incomplete ablation[21] and in the last case asymptomatic hemorrhage along the trajectory tract[21]

Our cavernoma case had a radiological outcome with the almost complete disappearance of the lesion during the follow-up. The major complication (unilateral hearing loss) was probably due to the proximity of the auditory pathways to the ablation area. More cases and a longer period of follow-up are required to support the claims of long-lasting symptom relief, hemorrhage-free survival, and disease recurrence.

Posterior Fossa MRI-Guided Laser Interstitial Thermal Therapy: Complications

Both thermal ablation (due to hyperthermia, post-ablation edema, or ablation-induced bleeding) and stereotactic laser insertion might cause intraoperative or postoperative complications.

In their recent systematic review, Sahabi and colleagues[1] reported procedure-related complications, usually including new neurologic deficits, in approximately 14.5% (19/131 patients) who underwent MRgLITT in the posterior fossa. In most cases, neurologic impairments improved either naturally or in conjunction with steroid therapy and rehabilitation, usually within six months.

The analysis of the data shows that the proximity of the lesion to the cranial nerves' nuclei is the primary determinant in the onset of new neurological deficit after the LITT. Therefore, patients with brainstem lesions had a higher risk of problems, whereas ablation of the cerebellum had a lower risk.

Patients with complications showed lower postablation-to-preablation tumor volume ratios. It is therefore important to acquire and integrate

functional studies (tractography, connectomics) in the preoperative planning in an anatomically and functionally dense area such as the posterior fossa.

Robot-guided MRgLITT can also provide several benefits, including those associated with more precise insertion of laser fibers, smaller incisions, and shorter hospital stays.

To obtain better results, a technological improvement is also desirable with the possibility of a 3D real-time monitoring, and the possibility of better modulating the limits of thermal ablation or of angulating the laser fiber.

SUMMARY

Minimally invasive techniques like MRgLITT will not completely replace open surgical techniques, but they will complement them and offer alternate therapeutic approaches in some selected pediatric patients. Although the minimally invasive nature of LITT makes it appealing to patients, parents, and neurosurgeons, research is still ongoing into how LITT compares to more conventional techniques in terms of safety and clinical outcome. Given the region's proximity to vital structures, care must be taken to prevent damage to nearby structures. It is crucial to be aware of these consequences, especially for benign diseases, as they may affect the quality of life after LITT.

DISCLOSURE

The authors have nothing to disclose.

CLINICS CARE POINTS

> Currently, there are no treatment recommendations for laser interstitial thermal therapy of the pediatric posterior fossa due to a limited pool of data. Objectives of future works is to establish efficacy and safety profile of posterior fossa MRI-guided laser interstitial thermal treatment in children in terms of degree of tumor ablation, control of local tumor and complication's rate.

SUPPLEMENTARY DATA

Supplementary data related to this article can be found online at https://doi.org/10.1016/j.nec.2022.11.002.

REFERENCES

1. Sabahi M, Bordes SJ, Najera E, et al. Laser interstitial thermal therapy for posterior fossa lesions: a

systematic review and analysis of multi-institutional outcomes. Cancers (Basel) 2022;14(2):456.

2. Lin CT, Riva-Cambrin JK. Management of posterior fossa tumors and hydrocephalus in children: a review. Childs Nerv Syst 2015;31:1781–9.

3. Picariello S, Spennato P, Roth J, et al. Posterior fossa tumours in the first year of life: a two-centre retrospective study. Diagnostics (Basel) 2022;12(3):635.

4. Onorini N, Spennato P, Orlando V, et al. The clinical and prognostic impact of the choice of surgical approach to fourth ventricular tumors in a single-center, single-surgeon cohort of 92 consecutive pediatric patients. Front Oncol 2022;12:821738.

5. Candela-Cantó S, Muchart J, Ramírez-Camacho A, et al. Robot-assisted, real-time, MRI-guided laser interstitial thermal therapy for pediatric patients with hypothalamic hamartoma: surgical technique, pitfalls, and initial results. J Neurosurg Pediatr 2022;29(6):681–92.

6. Hect JL, Alattar AA, Harford EE, et al. Stereotactic laser interstitial thermal therapy for the treatment of pediatric drug-resistant epilepsy: indications, techniques, and safety. Childs Nerv Syst 2022;38(5):961–70.

7. Bozinov O, Yang Y, Oertel M, et al. Laser interstitial thermal therapy in gliomas. Cancer Lett 2020;474:151–7.

8. Riordan M, Tovar-Spinoza Z. Laser induced thermal therapy (LITT) for pediatric brain tumors: case-based review. Transl Pediatr 2014;3(3):229–35.

9. Patel PD, Ashraf O, Danish SF. Magnetic resonance-guided laser interstitial thermal therapy for brainstem pathologies. World Neurosurg 2022;161:e80–9.

10. Traylor JI, Patel R, Habib A, et al. Laser interstitial thermal therapy to the posterior fossa: challenges and nuances. World Neurosurg 2019;132:e124–32.

11. Borghei-Razavi H, Koech H, Sharma M, et al. Laser interstitial thermal therapy for posterior fossa lesions: an initial experience. World Neurosurg 2018;117:e146–53.

12. Ashraf O, Arzumanov G, Luther E, et al. Magnetic resonance-guided laser interstitial thermal therapy for posterior fossa neoplasms. J Neurooncol 2020;149(3):533–42.

13. Formisano M, Iuppariello L, Mirone G. et al. "3D Printed Anatomical Model for Surgical Planning: a Pediatric Hospital Experience," 2021 International Conference on e-Health and Bioengineering (EHB), 2021, pp. 1-4

14. Saenz A, Singh J, Gan HW, et al. A novel technique for frame-based MR-guided laser ablation in an infant. Childs Nerv Syst 2022. https://doi.org/10.1007/s00381-022-05616-2.

15. Gupta N. A modification of the Mayfield horseshoe headrest allowing pin fixation and cranial immobilization in infants and young children. Neurosurgery 2006;58(1 Suppl):ONS-E181 [discussion: ONS-E181].

16. Lee M, Rezai AR, Chou J. Depressed skull fractures in children secondary to skull clamp fixation devices. Pediatr Neurosurg 1994;21:174–7.

17. Lee JJ, Clarke D, Hoverson E, et al. MRI-guided laser interstitial thermal therapy using the Visualase system and Navigus frameless stereotaxy in an infant: technical case report. J Neurosurg Pediatr 2021;1–4.

18. Dadey DY, Kamath AA, Smyth MD, et al. Utilizing personalized stereotactic frames for laser interstitial thermal ablation of posterior fossa and mesiotemporal brain lesions: a single-institution series. Neurosurg Focus 2016;41(4):E4.

19. Tovar-Spinoza Z, Choi H. Magnetic resonance-guided laser interstitial thermal therapy: report of a series of pediatric brain tumors. J Neurosurg Pediatr 2016;17(6):723–33.

20. Willie JT, Malcolm JG, Stern MA, et al. Safety and effectiveness of stereotactic laser ablation for epileptogenic cerebral cavernous malformations. Epilepsia 2019;60(2):220–32.

21. Malcolm JG, Douglas JM, Greven A, et al. Feasibility and morbidity of magnetic resonance imaging-guided stereotactic laser ablation of deep cerebral cavernous malformations: a report of 4 cases. Neurosurgery 2021;89(4):635–44.

22. Lawrence JD, Rehman A, Lee M. Treatment of a pontine cavernoma with laser interstitial thermal therapy: case report. J Neurol Surg B Skull Base 2021;82(S 02):P177.

23. Gamboa NT, Karsy M, Iyer RR, et al. Stereotactic laser interstitial thermal therapy for brainstem cavernous malformations: two preliminary cases. Acta Neurochir 2020;162:1771–5.

24. Yousefi O, Sabahi M, Malcolm J, et al. Laser interstitial thermal therapy for cavernous malformations: a systematic review. Front Surg 2022;9:887329.

Awake Laser Ablation with Continuous Neuropsychological Testing During Treatment of Brain Tumors and Epilepsy

Silas Haahr Nielsen, MD[a], Jane Skjøth-Rasmussen, MD, PhD[a],
Signe Delin Moldrup, MSc, Clinical neuropsychologist[a],
Christina Malling Engelmann, MSc, Clinical neuropsychologist[b,1],
Bo Jespersen, MD[a], Rune Rasmussen, MD, PhD[a,*]

KEYWORDS

• LITT • Mapping • Awake surgery • Neuropsychology

KEY POINTS

- Laser interstitial thermal therapy (LITT) in the awake patient is feasible and safe.
- Continuous neurologic evaluation during laser ablation can guide perioperative decisions.
- In our experience, the awake LITT workflow is valuable in achieving maximal safe ablation.
- If no involvement of dura mater, the patient feels no pain during laser ablation.

INTRODUCTION

MR-guided laser interstitial thermal therapy (LITT) is an emerging minimally invasive neurosurgical technique in the treatment of drug-resistant epilepsy, brain tumors and radiation necrosis.[1–4] LITT is typically performed with the patient under general anesthesia. Here, we present a novel approach to perform LITT in the awake patient using continuous neuropsychological monitoring.

Stereotactic accuracy, near real-time monitoring of the ablative lesion with thermal maps and thermal damage estimate maps as well as the rapid fall of light energy in biological tissue[5] provides the ability to achieve steep borders to the surrounding brain tissue. This has led to the usage of LITT to treat lesions adjacent to eloquent brain areas and subcortical fiber tracts independent of depth in the brain. However, treatment with LITT is not without surgical risks, with the most common complications being temporary and permanent neurological deficits (8.82%–35.5% and 2.17%–7.14%, respectively[6]). Performing LITT in the awake patient with continuous neuropsychological evaluation may help to preserve neurologic function.

To our knowledge, only 2 studies have so far described the use of LITT in the awake patient.

In 2018, Laurent and colleagues[7] from University of Florida described a novel workflow for LITT implementation in 10 awake patients with recurrent primary brain tumors using 3-dimensional-printed patient-specific facemasks for stereotactic placement of the laser probe and noninvasive immobilization of patients. The treatment was performed in the diagnostic MRI suite using the Neuroblate system (Monteris medical, Minnetonka, MN, USA). Patients were administered low doses of

[a] Department of Neurosurgery, Rigshospitalet, Entrance 8, 6th Floor, Inge Lehmanns Vej 8, 2100, Copenhagen East, Denmark; [b] Center for Neurorehabilitation, Lions Kollegiet, Copenhagen, Denmark
[1] Entrance 8, 6th floor, Inge Lehmanns Vej 8, 2100 Copenhagen East.
* Corresponding author.
E-mail address: rune.rasmussen@regionh.dk

Neurosurg Clin N Am 34 (2023) 239–245
https://doi.org/10.1016/j.nec.2022.11.003
1042-3680/23/© 2022 Elsevier Inc. All rights reserved.

oral narcotics for pain control. For patients with lesions in eloquent areas, a targeted neurological exam was performed intermittently once the thermal treatment field reached approximately 80% of the tumor volume. They concluded that LITT can be delivered safely and accurately in the awake patient using customized facemasks.

By their experience, the benefits of awake LITT are avoiding general anesthesia exposure to patients, reduction in operative time and length of in-hospital stay, and a reduction in postablation neurological deficits. A drawback with this approach is that the production of customized facemasks increases the preoperative preparation time and introduces additional costs.

In 2020, Hajtovic and colleagues[8] from New York University described an awake LITT workflow with conventional head-fixation in the MRI. They described the treatment of 6 patients with brain tumors who underwent awake LITT with 3 different workflows, because of a change in the institution's facilities and the installation of an intraoperative MRI for the last 2 cases. The patients were mildly sedated using dexmedetomidine in all patients, propofol in 4 patients, remifentanil in 3 patients, and ketamine in 3 patients. The neurological status was intermittently assessed approximately every 5 minutes during the ablation. They found that awake LITT in eloquent brain areas is safe and feasible and useful in preventing neurological deficits.

Here, we present a novel workflow for LITT in the awake patient that capitalizes on our experience from awake brain mapping. In contrast to the previous published studies, we propose an awake LITT workflow with neuropsychological assistance and continuous neurologic evaluation, no sedation during laser ablation and head-fixation in an MRI-compatible head-ring. Moreover, we describe this workflow for the treatment of both tumors and epilepsy.

METHOD
Equipment

- Radionics cosman–roberts–wells (CRW) frame with MRI-compatible UCHRA head-ring (Universal Compact Head Ring)
- Intraoperative MRI GE SIGNA Artist 1.5 Tesla
- BrainLab AIRO Mobile computed tomography (CT) scanner
- MRI-compatible frame-holder from ClearPoint
- Medtronic Visualase MRI-guided laser ablation system

Patient Selection

- If the target is eligible for LITT treatment and located near eloquent cortical structures or subcortical fiber tracts the awake treatment workflow is suggested. Patients with brain tumors and epilepsy patients are eligible for awake LITT.

WORKFLOW
Preparation

- Preoperative MRI
- Trajectory planning using BrainLab Elements
- Conversation with the neurosurgeon performing the LITT procedure
- Preoperative interview and neurocognitive testing with the neuropsychologist
- The purpose of the preoperative neuropsychological testing is not to make a standard neuropsychological assessment but to obtain a baseline of the relevant motor, sensor, and cognitive functions. Furthermore, the patient and relatives are informed in detail about the procedure and possible deficits both during and after the treatment. It is underlined, that neurological and neuropsychological deficits cannot be prevented completely but that it might be limited compared with treatment in general anesthesia

In the operation room

- Most patients are initially mildly sedated using intravenous propofol
- A bladder catheter is inserted
- The patient is placed in the MRI-compatible head-ring with local anesthesia in the skin at the pin insertion sites
- A CT-scan is obtained with the CT localizer frame (BRWLF)
- The preoperative MRI-scan and the perioperative CT-scan is fused using BrainLab Elements, and stereotactic coordinates for the placement of the laser catheter is obtained
- The CRW stereotactic frame is mounted to the MRI-compatible head-ring
- Stab incision in the skin
- A 3.2-mm burr hole in skull
- Dura puncture
- The laser catheter is placed using the Visualase skull bolt
- Correct placement of the laser catheter is verified using a CT-scan
- The patient is moved to the MRI table, and the MRI-compatible head-ring from CRW is mounted to the MRI-compatible frame-holder from ClearPoint using strips (**Fig. 1**)
- The patient is then moved to the MRI that is located next to the operation room

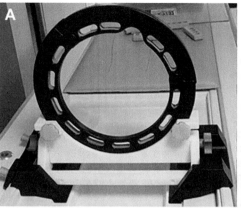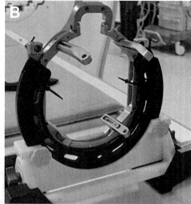

Fig. 1. MRI-compatible head-ring (*B*) mounted to the MRI-compatible frame-holder (*A*) using strips.

In the MRI

- A preoperative MRI T1 is performed. In patients with malignant tumors half-dose Gadolinium-based contrast is given.
- The neuropsychologist is located next to the patient (**Fig. 2**) while in the MRI-scanner and continuously evaluating neurologic function of the patient.
- In ablations near fiber tracts, the tissue is heated to 45° for 30 to 60 seconds, treatment is paused, and a focused neurologic and neuropsychological examination is performed.

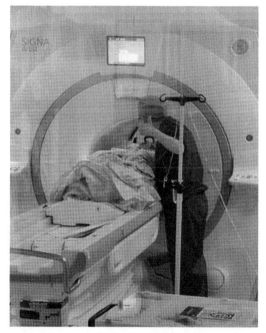

Fig. 2. Neuropsychologist, Christina Malling Engelmann, continuous testing neurologic function inside the MRI-room.

- Perioperative surgical decisions of ablation diameter and number of retractions are made using information of the patient's neurological status and agreements with the patient obtained preoperatively.
- A postoperative MRI T1 is performed. In patients with malignant tumors the second half-dose Gadolinium-based contrast is given.

Neuropsychological testing

- Depending on location relevant brain functions are monitored but there are limitations of the narrow MRI gantry and noise during imaging sessions.
- Continuous evaluation of motor function and visual fields is achievable during laser ablation (the latter by moving a nonmagnetic stick above the patients' head and asking the patient to squint when they no longer see the stick); however, higher cognitive functions are not possible to test during the ablation due to noise from the MRI.
- In between sessions, other functions can be tested, for instance, sensation, working memory, and language-functions (such as spontaneous speech, articulation, naming, sentence-repetition, comprehension). Furthermore, the neuropsychologist can make sure that the patient is emotionally well and/or provide emotional support.
- The neuropsychologist continuously communicates with the surgeon outside the MR suite using hand-gestures. Thumbs up hand-gesture for continued ablation and time out hand-gesture for stop ablation.

Postablation in the operation room

- Removal of laser catheter and head-ring.
- Single suture in the skin.

CASE

Background: A 28-year-old woman with recurrent frontotemporal and insular diffuse astrocytoma (WHO grading 2, isocitrate dehydrogenase 1 mutation, methylation of the O^6-methylguanine-DNA methyl-transferase gene promoter). She previously has had 2 awake craniotomies with mapping. After the first operation, she suffered from a mild left-sided facial palsy and less visual attention to the left. Furthermore, she had left-sided focal seizures (5–10 per month) and some generalized seizures. Besides this, she was well functioning and able to work full time. The MRI revealed a remnant posteriorly in the insular region on the right-side (**Fig. 3**A). Because of a strong patient wish, we choose to reduce the tumor burden with awake LITT. An agreement was made with the patient to abort treatment if neurologic deterioration occurred during laser ablation.

Neuropsychologial testing: The tumor was located posteriorly in the insula near the corticospinal tracts (CSTs) and the superior longitudinal fasciculus (SLF) II and III. During laser ablation, the patient was continuously tested for left hand, leg, and facial movements (CST). In between treatment sessions, when there was no noise from the MRI, the patient was screened for self-experience (body sensation, autonomous reaction–insula), visual attention and reading (SLF II and III), perception of touch by tactile stimulation (insula and CST), working memory (insula), and vocal quality and articulation (CST, insula, and SLF II).

Procedure: The patient was awake during the entire treatment with local anesthesia in the skin, analgesia with paracetamol and mild sedation with propofol during head fixation and placement of the laser catheter. The laser catheter was placed through the prefrontal region and into the posterior part of the insula. The final placement of the laser catheter on the perioperative CT-scan was 1 mm off the intended target. During the treatment, the patient experienced no pain, nausea, or discomfort. She was very cooperative and able to fulfill the tasks. Initially, the center of the tumor was ablated. Next, the catheter was pushed further in, and the deep part of the tumor was ablated. Finally, the catheter was retracted, and the upper part of the tumor was ablated. During the final ablation (**Fig. 4**), the patient had worsening of her preexisting facial palsy, and we chose to abort further treatment. The temperature at the presumed location of the CSTs was 44°C to 47°C for less than 30 seconds.

Follow-up: Postoperatively she continued to have a discrete worsening of the facial palsy. During the following weeks, the palsy gradually remitted. Besides this, she did not have any cognitive decline, the seizure frequency decreased substantially, and we had obtained local control on the 3-month follow-up MRI (**Fig. 3**B and C). However, in the following months after treatment, she was not able to work full-time (25 hours weekly) because of intermittent headache and tiredness.

DISCUSSION

To date, 5 patients with epilepsy and 4 patients with brain tumors have been treated with awake LITT at our center. It is our initial experience that LITT in the awake patient with continuous testing of neurological function is feasible, safe, and useful in preventing neurological deficits. In patients where deterioration in neurological function is detected early during ablation, the ablation can be aborted to avoid further loss of function as done in 3 of our cases. Furthermore, the initial loss of function might be reversible at temperatures below cell kill intensity (10–30 minutes at 43°C[5,9–14]). This even opens up the possibility of using controlled heating below the threshold for permanent tissue damage to be used as a mapping function.

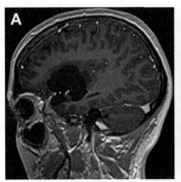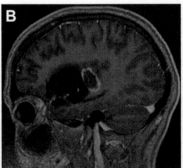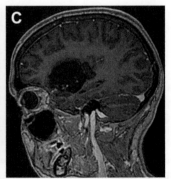

Fig. 3. (*A*) Preoperative MRI T1 with contrast. (*B*) Early postoperative MRI T1 with contrast. (*C*) 3 months follow-up MRI T1 with contrast.

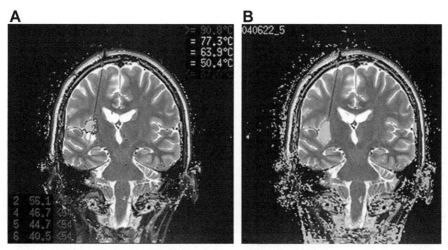

Fig. 4. (*A*) Heat map. (*B*) Irreversible estimated damage map during laser ablation. Temperature at markers located on the CST (4, 5, and 6) revealed a temperature from 44.7°C to 46.7°C.

In the awake LITT workflow, the clinician faces similar challenges as in awake craniotomy with brain mapping. It is challenging to respond to the continuous information about the neurological status and how this should affect treatment decisions. Hence, it is of utmost importance to consider multiple scenarios and discuss these with the patient before operation. Should we proceed to ablate the entire tumor despite minor neurological deficits? How much function loss is acceptable to the patient? Should we abort the ablation even if only part of the tumor has been treated? These decisions depend on patient wishes, severity of the neurological deficit, pathologic condition treated, evidence level for surgery, and the physician's and the team's experience with LITT and awake surgery. Despite the challenges, it is our experience that awake LITT offers an additional layer of protection for the patient and, in some cases, even allows us to be more radical in our treatments. If a tumor near an eloquent area is treated and the patient is still neurologically intact when most of the tumor is ablated, this information can provide the surgeon with confidence to make a supramarginal ablation.

By our experience, the awake LITT workflow does not increase the procedural time. Average procedural time is 4 hours for awake LITT versus an average procedural time of 4 hours and 20 minutes in 40 LITT treatments performed with the patients under general anesthesia. The time used for comforting and testing the patient is matched by the time saved from avoiding endotracheal intubation. Avoidance of the risk associated with endotracheal intubation and general anesthesia is an advantage of the awake LITT workflow. This is especially an advantage for centers without an intraoperative MRI, and therefore, they are required to transport the patient from the operation room to the diagnostic MRI. Additional benefits are easier postoperative observation and possible cost/benefit increase.

Having an existing working setup for awake craniotomy has been an advantage at our center because this setup could be transferred to the awake LITT setup. Centers considering awake LITT could benefit from using their own setup. Having an experienced dedicated professional to perform the continuous neurological evaluation is important. Moreover, this person adds substantially to patient comfort and satisfaction because they will follow the patient before, during, and after treatment.

Performing the treatment with the patient awake also introduces risks. The near real-time updated thermal maps require no head movement during ablation since MRI-thermography assumes that the spatial location of the patient's head is fixed inside the MRI. Accidental patient movement inside the MRI is not automatically detected by the software using the Visualase System from Medtronic and can compromise treatment safety. Head fixation is therefore paramount. Head-fixation using the MR-compatible head-ring combined with the frame-holder attached to the MRI bed provides a rigid head-fixation and is therefore sufficient. Furthermore, head-fixation in the MRI-compatible head-ring allows for almost unlimited placement of the laser catheter while keeping the patient in supine position in the MRI that enables neurological testing, and there is no need to refixate the head after placement of the LITT catheter. A drawback to our approach is the need of a somewhat improvised solution for attaching the 2 head holders using plastic strips. Commercial frame holders for MRI tables are probably available. It has previously been described that awake LITT without head fixation is possible[8] as a salvage solution. However, in our experience, this should be avoided entirely because the patient is awake and answers commands.

Awake LITT requires a cooperative patient that is able to endure fixation in a head-ring for several hours as well as neurological testing inside the MRI. Patient pain and discomfort in the operating room or during laser ablation is a risk. However, we have not had any patients reporting severe discomfort during treatment. Pain during laser ablation is previously reported[7,8] when ablating lesions near dura mater. None of our patients has reported pain during laser ablation; however, we have had no treatments close to dura. Ablations involving brain parenchyma did not produce pain. However, a cold feeling from the salt-water cooled catheter at skin level has been reported by a few patients.

The previously published studies have not treated patients with epilepsy as the primary indication. In theory, there is a risk of inducing a seizure by heating the assumed epileptic focus. Again, a thorough planning of this scenario is important. Antiepileptic drugs should be prepared together with a well-organized evacuation plan. So far, we have not experienced any seizures during awake LITT treatments.

Although neuropsychological testing can help to minimize neurological deficit, it is important to inform the patient that it does not guarantee that neurological deficits can be avoided entirely. Even if the patient during awake treatment is neurological intact, postablation neurological deterioration can occur in the following days to weeks after treatment, presumably due to edema, enlargement of the ablation cavity or delayed cell death.

However, most of the delayed neurological deficits will be reversible and treatment with corticosteroids should be considered.[8]

The awake LITT workflow can be applied to most LITT treatments to help minimize neurological deficits; avoid general anesthesia; and reduce procedural time, postoperative observation, and length of in-hospital stay. The workflow can be further improved with an MRI-compatible communication system with noise reduction, projection of visual stimuli to the patient inside the MRI for improved neuropsychological testing and head-fixation without the need of improvised solutions with plastic strips.

CLINICS CARE POINTS

- The main points of the workflow are easily implementable but to adapt the suggested workflow LITT Centers must take advantage of their own setup, equipment, and personnel.

- The stereotactic frame serves for both catheter placement and rigid fixation during MRI.

- Awake LITT surgery introduces similar dilemmas and challenges as in awake craniotomies with mapping. Make an agreement with the patient regarding when to stop the ablation.

- Conventional head-fixation using an MRI compatible head-ring in the MRI is feasible for awake LITT with continuous neurological testing with the patient in supine position.

- Awake LITT can provide the surgeon with valuable information during laser ablation that helps in preserving neurological function.

DISCLOSURE

None.

ACKNOWLEDGMENTS

The project is funded by the Danish Comprehensive Cancer Center (DCCC) Brain Tumor Center. We wish to thank Christine Sølling and Martin Kryspin Sørensen from Department of Neuroanaesthesiology, Copenhagen University Hospital for assisting in developing the awake patient workflow.

REFERENCES

1. Kim AH, Tatter S, Rao G, et al. Laser Ablation of Abnormal Neurological Tissue Using Robotic Neuro-Blate System (LAANTERN): 12-Month Outcomes and Quality of Life After Brain Tumor Ablation. Neurosurgery 2020;87(3):E338–46.
2. Munoz-Casabella A, Alvi MA, Rahman M, et al. Laser Interstitial Thermal Therapy for Recurrent Glioblastoma: Pooled Analyses of Available Literature. World Neurosurg 2021;153:91–7.e1.
3. Wu C, Schwalb JM, Rosenow JM, et al. The American Society for Stereotactic and Functional Neurosurgery Position Statement on Laser Interstitial Thermal Therapy for the Treatment of Drug-Resistant Epilepsy. Neurosurgery 2022;90(2): 155–60.

4. Ahluwalia M, Barnett GH, Deng D, et al. Laser ablation after stereotactic radiosurgery: a multicenter prospective study in patients with metastatic brain tumors and radiation necrosis. J Neurosurg 2018; 130(3):804–11.

5. McNichols RJ, Gowda A, Kangasniemi M, et al. MR thermometry-based feedback control of laser interstitial thermal therapy at 980 nm. Lasers Surg Med 2004;34(1):48–55.

6. Holste KG, Orringer DA. Laser interstitial thermal therapy. Neurooncol Adv 2019;2(1):vdz035.

7. Laurent D, Oliveria SF, Shang M, et al. Techniques to ensure accurate targeting for delivery of awake laser interstitial thermotherapy. Oper Neurosurg (Hagerstown) 2018;15(4):454–60.

8. Hajtovic S, Mogilner A, Ard J, et al. Awake Laser Ablation for Patients With Tumors in Eloquent Brain Areas: Operative Technique and Case Series. Cureus 2020;12(12):e12186.

9. Ghanouni P, Pauly KB, Elias WJ, et al. Transcranial MRI-Guided Focused Ultrasound: A Review of the Technologic and Neurologic Applications. AJR Am J Roentgenol 2015;205(1):150–9.

10. Rieke V, Butts Pauly K. MR thermometry. J Magn Reson Imaging 2008;27(2):376–90.

11. Chang IA. Considerations for thermal injury analysis for RF ablation devices. Open Biomed Eng J 2010;4: 3–12.

12. Dewhirst MW, Viglianti BL, Lora-Michiels M, et al. Basic principles of thermal dosimetry and thermal thresholds for tissue damage from hyperthermia. Int J Hyperthermia 2003;19(3):267–94.

13. Sminia P, Haveman J, Ongerboer de Visser BW. What is a safe heat dose which can be applied to normal brain tissue? Int J Hyperthermia 1989;5(1): 115–7.

14. Haveman J, Sminia P, Wondergem J, et al. Effects of hyperthermia on the central nervous system: what was learnt from animal studies? Int J Hyperthermia 2005;21(5):473–87.

Laser Interstitial Thermal Therapy for Epilepsy

Jamie J. Van Gompel, MD[a],*, David B. Burkholder, MD[b], Jonathon J. Parker, MD, PhD[c], Sangeet S. Grewal, MD[d], Erik H. Middlebrooks, MD[e], Vance T. Lehman, MD[f], Kai J. Miller, MD, PhD[a], Eva C. Alden, PhD[g], Timothy J. Kaufmann, MD, MS[f]

KEYWORDS

- Laser interstitial thermal therapy (LITT) • Epilepsy • Minimally invasive

KEY POINTS

- Laser interstitial thermal therapy (LITT) has a diverse use in epilepsy.
- Offers a minimally invasive option attempting to limit approach-related comorbidity.
- Long-term data are yet lacking compared with open surgical data.

INTRODUCTION

In recent years, laser interstitial thermal therapy (LITT) has emerged as an alternative to open surgery for many patients with drug-resistant epilepsy or neoplasm. Increasing neurosurgeon experience is creating potential for more widespread implementation for epilepsy management. The basic physical premise is that high-density light is converted to heat energy within the tissue of a confined and controllable region, monitored with magnetic resonance thermometry.

Advantages of LITT include a less-invasive approach with faster recovery, increased tissue preservation, the potential to recruit patients who might decline open surgery, and preserved ability to re-treat with either LITT or open surgery if needed. LITT may be particularly useful for areas of relatively high surgical risk or complexity, such as the insular targets. Nonetheless, surgical outcomes remain superior for some indications, and there is relatively little prospective or long-term data. For most indications, the preponderant publications remain based on small case series.

Use for treating epilepsy is unique in that the primary treatment endpoint may be either complete ablation of a lesion or functional disconnection. Specific focal lesions are numerous and include malformations of cortical development, low-grade neoplasms such as dysembryoplastic neuroepithelial tumor, hypothalamic hamartoma (HH), tubers, cavernous malformations, and temporal lobe encephaloceles. Functional disconnection is sought with temporal lobe epilepsy (TLE; either nonlesional or with mesial temporal lobe sclerosis [MTS]), corpus callosotomy, stereotactic electroencephalogram (sEEG)-positive/MRI-negative seizures, and encephalomalacia-related seizures.

A key consideration is that the treatment is ideally the result of a rigorous multidisciplinary evaluation. Neurologists serve a central role in the initial diagnosis, medical treatment optimization, semiology evaluation, and EEG interpretation. Neuroradiologists optimize and tailor anatomic and functional imaging protocols for diagnosis and procedure planning. Neurosurgeons synthesize this information to formulate and offer

[a] Department of Neurosurgery Mayo Clinic, 200 First street, SouthWest, Rochester, MN 55905, USA; [b] Department of Neurology, Division of epilepsy, Mayo Clinic, 200 First street, SouthWest, Rochester, MN 55905, USA; [c] Department of Neurosurgery Mayo Clinic, 13400 East Shea Boulevard, Scottsdale, AZ 85259, USA; [d] Department of Neurosurgery Mayo Clinic, 4500 San Pablo Road S Building 3-310, Jacksonville, FL 32224, USA; [e] Department of Radiology Mayo Clinic, 4500 San Pablo Road S Building 3-310, Jacksonville, FL 32224; [f] Department of Radiology Mayo Clinic, 200 First street, SouthWest, Rochester, MN 55905, USA; [g] Department of Psychiatry Mayo Clinic, 200 First street, SouthWest, Rochester, MN 55905, USA
* Corresponding author.
E-mail address: Vangompel.jamie@mayo.edu

Neurosurg Clin N Am 34 (2023) 247–257
https://doi.org/10.1016/j.nec.2022.11.005
1042-3680/23/© 2022 Elsevier Inc. All rights reserved.

appropriate surgical treatment options. At our institution, complex cases are evaluated for procedure candidacy with a full review of all pertinent information by a multidisciplinary committee. A team approach during and after the procedure was also implemented. This article will review the key technical, clinical, radiologic, and neurosurgical considerations for LITT management of epilepsy, emphasizing the advantages of a multidisciplinary approach.

Background

Thermal ablation with resultant necrosis and cytoreduction is the primary mechanism used for LITT for epilepsy. However, other potential mechanisms are being explored for LITT more broadly, such as blood–brain barrier opening effects. According to the Arrhenius equation, tissue necrosis depends on temperature and time. In brief, necrosis does not occur less than 43°C and is instantaneous at 60°C. At 100°C, water vaporization and carbonization can result in tissue cavitation, referred to as a "steam event."

Near real-time MR thermometry based on temperature-dependent features of MRI signal, typically with proton resonance frequency shift imaging,[1] permits the creation of heat maps and estimated cell damage maps during the procedure. Temperature-limit markers are strategically placed to avoid damage to nearby critical structures and to prevent vaporization in the hottest region.

Laser fibers are produced by 2 major vendors, each with unique designs, placement methods, ablation patterns, and cooling methods. These can be placed by a variety of standard stereotactic techniques. Also varying by vendor, laser applicators are available with varying diameters, laser wavelength, diffusing tip length, and power levels. Optical fiber diffusing tips are also available in isotropic or directional variants depending on the vendor. Specifics of available LITT equipment continue to evolve. Trajectory planning and placement are the key steps to a technically successful procedure.

DISCUSSION
Temporal Lobe Epilepsy—Lesional

TLE is one of the most common variants of focal epilepsy. Anterior temporal lobectomy (ATL) was reported as a surgical option in treating medically refractory temporal lobe epilepsy in 1950. Many still consider this the gold standard surgical treatment of TLE.[2] As techniques progressed, selective amygdalohippocampectomy was popularized for mesial temporal lobe epilepsy (MTLE) treatment. Compared with ATL, a selective amygdalohippocampectomy

leads to seizure-free outcomes that are within 10% of seizure-free rates of ATL.[3] However, visual field and verbal memory deficits with ATL seem greater than selective amygdalohippocampectomy (43% vs 31%).[4] The potential for effectiveness balances seizure freedom with the risk of "collateral damage" incurred by neocortical resection of the anterior temporal lobe.[5] MTS is the most common pathologic condition in patients with MTLE.[6–10] For treating patients with MTLE, many centers have transitioned from ATL and selective amygdalohippocampectomy to LITT. The surgical approach is typically performed by occipital insertion of the LITT catheter following an extraventricular trajectory along the long axis of the hippocampal formation (**Fig. 1** Hippo). Following this, the hippocampus and amygdala ablation is performed with concomitant MRI monitoring. Currently, there is no class I evidence to compare the efficacy and complication rates observed with selective laser amygdalohippocampectomy (SLAH) and ATL. However, there is currently enrolling a Medtronic Industry Sponsored study, Stereotactic Laser Ablation for Temporal lobe Epilepsy (SLATE), to provide level one evidence. Available literature from retrospective case series studies (Class III data) suggest an efficacy rate of SLAH that is comparable but slightly less than outcomes seen after ATL (38%–70%), whereas surgical complication rates for SLAH that are less than that for ATL.[11–22] Studies have suggested that LITT has resulted in a lower rate of neuropsychological deficits compared with traditional approaches. However, there may be no significant difference in postoperative visual field deficits.[13,20–24] A large analysis of 234 patients undergoing MRgLITT at multiple institutions found a hemorrhage rate of 1.5% with a rate of persistent neurological complications in 11% of patients (majority visual field deficits).[25] Studies have performed a volumetric analysis of patients undergoing MRgLITT and found no correlation between total ablation volume and seizure outcome. However, in patients with persistent seizures following SLAH, there may be an association of mesial hippocampal head sparing with persistent disabling seizures.[13,20,21] As there has been no significant correlation between length of ablation or volume of ablation and seizure freedom, there remains some controversy as to the ideal ablation. Depending on the curvature of the mesial temporal lobe structures, an adequate ablation could require multiple trajectories, as has been suggested by some studies.

Nonlesional temporal lobe epilepsy

It is well recognized that nonlesional epilepsy has consistently demonstrated worse surgical outcomes than lesional epilepsy, making this an important area for improvement in our diagnostic

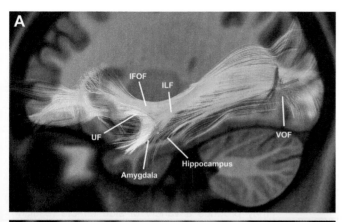

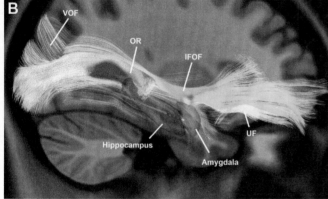

Fig. 1. hippo: T1-weighted sagittal images with MR tractography demonstrating the relevant tract anatomy for LITT ablation of the amygdalohippocampus. (*A*) Lateral projection showing the relationship of the inferior fronto-occipital fasciculus (IFOF; cyan), uncinate fasciculus (UF; yellow), inferior longitudinal fasciculus (ILF; green), and vertical occipital fasciculus (VOF; purple), which lie lateral to the hippocampus (red) and amygdala (blue). The UF, IFOF, and ILF may be transgressed in open approaches to resection the amygdala and hippocampus with potential for neurological consequence. (*B*) Medial projection also reveals the close association of these tracts plus the optic radiations (OR; light orange). The laser trajectory typically traverses these tracts but limits injury as opposed to open resection.

and surgical approaches.[26] The use of LITT as a surgical ablation strategy for epilepsy patients without an identifiable lesion detected on MRI is increasingly used because of lower morbidity than open resection. However, this technique requires a precise sEEG-mapped seizure onset to target in most cases. Further, the optimal extent of ablation around an sEEG-mapped seizure onset zone is unknown.

Laser ablation of the mesial temporal structures provides the largest reported experience with LITT for nonlesional epilepsy. Moreover, the reported rate of seizure freedom across studies using stereotactic laser amygdalohippocampectomy (SLAH) in cases without MTS is highly variable, ranging from 30% to 58%. In the largest series of SLAH procedures (n = 234 patients), Wu and colleagues[25] found no significant differences in seizure freedom rate in those with imaging evidence of hippocampal sclerosis compared with those without after 24 months of follow-up. Additionally, across all patients, invasive intracranial monitoring was not associated with an improvement in seizure outcome, although the rate of intracranial monitoring in nonhippocampal sclerosis patients was not separately reported. In a

large single institution series of 58 SLAH patients, only 5/15 (33%) patients without MTS achieved Engel I outcomes after at least 12 months of follow-up.[27] This reported outcome was comparable to the 3 of 10 non-MTS patients achieving Engel I with mesial temporal LITT in a similar series of 21 patients.[28] The question of whether non-MTS patients who receive LITT benefit from preablation sEEG was recently addressed in a retrospective series. In this small study, Engel I was observed in 7 of 12 (58%) non-MTS mesial temporal lobe cases confirmed via sEEG, compared with 10 of 18 (56%) MTS cases with confirmatory sEEG, after 16 and 17 months of follow-up, respectively.[29] There is insufficient evidence to state that sEEG should be routinely used to tailor laser ablation whose semiology and scalp EEG are strongly right temporal in the nonlesional setting. However, both the Wu and colleagues[25] study of laser ablation and the recent Sone and colleagues[30] study reporting outcomes of open temporal lobectomy have associated the ablation and resection of specific hippocampal subregions with seizure outcome. Taken together, these data provide a conceptual basis by which sEEG could be used to interrogate tissue along the axis of the hippocampus to tailor a laser ablation. Further standardization and study of hippocampal amygdalar network sEEG before LITT will be needed to determine its ability to improve outcomes in nonlesional cases.

Extratemporal Nonlesional LITT

The efficacy of LITT for MRI-negative nonlesional epilepsy is sparsely reported outside of the temporal lobe. Further, there is a lack of systematic description of the sEEG electrographic onset patterns associated with targets for LITT therapy in nonlesional patients. Outside of the mesial temporal lobe, LITT targeting electrographic seizure onsets in the insula and cingulate gyrus has been commonly reported, although most series do not report differential outcomes by anatomic region of seizure onset. Recently, Gupta and colleagues[31] described 35 patients with extratemporal epilepsy targeted by LITT, and of these, 6 (17%) were nonlesional. In this series, 33% of nonlesional patients achieved Engel I compared with 63% of lesional patients. Uniquely, this study captured electrographic seizure onset patterns from sEEG data in a subset of 24 patients (lesional and nonlesional). The authors found that low-voltage fast activity, a well-characterized sensitive biomarker of the epileptic cortex, was associated with improved LITT outcomes in both lesional and nonlesional cases. In another series of 20 patients with 70% nonlesional onsets, a small subset of 7% underwent LITT treatment immediately after the sEEG mapping.[32] Of these nonlesional patients, 55% achieved Engel I or II seizure outcomes at a mean of 17.2 months postop. Finally, Gireesh and colleagues[33] reported a series of 9 patients with nonlesional epilepsy mapped to the insula or cingulate. Five patients had LITT targeted at the insula alone, 3 at the cingulate alone, and operculum. In this series, 6 of 9 patients (66%) had Engel I, 2 of 9 Engel II, and 1 of 9 Engel III, respectively. As reported outcomes vary widely for nonlesional LITT, different strategies for seizure onset zone determination by epileptologist and neurosurgeons, and the extent of ablation remain potential sources of variability that may underlie differences in outcome across series.

LITT within eloquent areas such as the insula or near motor areas has a substantial advantage. It is helpful to monitor critical and nearby structures with low-temperature limits, typically around 43°C. These limits serve as posts to limit lesioning temperatures within, for instance, the internal capsule, extreme capsule, or motor cortex. Accordingly, LITT has been a beneficial strategy for treating lesions such as cavernomas within

these regions alternatively mapped cortical areas by sEEG that would benefit by reducing approach-related morbidity.

HHs are discussed in a separate article and therefore, not covered here.

Corpus Callosotomy

Corpus callosotomy is reserved for the most extreme cases of intractable epilepsy. The procedure involves disconnecting the 2 hemispheres by sectioning the corpus callosum. It is effective specifically for the therapy for drop attack seizures, both tonic and atonic.[34] This disconnection may produce a variety of side effects resulting from the inability of the 2 sides of the brain to coordinate cognition, sensory, or motor processing.[35] To mitigate these adverse effects, partial callosotomies sparing the anterior or posterior portions of the corpus callosum have been developed.[36,37] When performing these via an open craniotomy, there may be morbidity beyond the expected collateral syndromes created by isolating the hemispheres due to transgressing the scalp, skull, and dura, retracting a cerebral hemisphere, and manipulating vasculature. The advent of LIIT allows the surgeon to perform the callosotomy under MRI guidance and attempt to minimize morbidity.

Using up to 4 laser trajectories separately targeting the genu, the anterior body of the corpus callosum, the posterior body of the corpus callosum and isthmus, the splenium, and a complete corpus callosotomy may be performed minimally invasively (**Fig. 2** CC).[38] Fewer trajectories are needed in many cases. However, this will depend on each patient's anatomy. A 2-trajectory laser intervention may effectively complete the full disconnection without reopening the prior craniotomy and dissecting through a scarred operative field for patients who have previously undergone a partial corpus callosotomy.[39]

Neurologist Role

The relationship between neurology and neurosurgery is arguably closer in epilepsy than in any other neurologic disease. Their combined efforts can dramatically change lives but individually neither can adequately care for patients with drug-resistant epilepsy. The neurologist's role is vital for setting up patients and neurosurgeons for success.

The most crucial role of the neurologist is confirming the diagnosis of epilepsy, the type of epilepsy, and for focal epilepsies, localizing seizure onset. Although this seems obvious, it bears mentioning as poor seizure characterization and

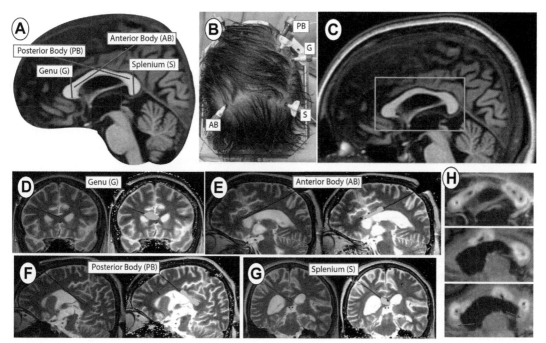

Fig. 2. *CC: A 4-trajectory approach to laser corpus callosotomy.* (*A*) Stereotypical trajectories for performing a complete interhemispheric disconnection, separately targeting the genu, anterior body, posterior body, and splenium. (*B*) Insertion sites for each trajectory. (*C*) The corpus callosum of the patient, with blue box indicating the location of the panels in (*H*). (*D*) Genu trajectory, showing the insertion on the left with the damage estimate in gold on the right. (*E*) As in (*D*) but for the anterior body trajectory. (*F*) As in (*D*) but for the posterior body trajectory. (*G*) As in (*D*) but for the splenium trajectory. (*H*) Postprocedure parasagittal sections through the corpus callosum, illustrating thermal ablation sites on a T1-weighted postcontrast MRI. Because ablations are ultimately produced in varying lateralities in the corpus callosum due to the angles of the trajectories required, multiple imaging views are needed to fully appreciate the complete ablation. Note that the most ventral aspect of both the genu and splenium are ablated at particular locations along the left-right traversal of their callosal fibers, though the nonablated portions of those same fibers will not have immediate postprocedure contrast enhancement (*red arrows*). This appearance could be misleading if the entire width of the corpus callosum is not evaluated.

localization prevent any chance of success with surgical interventions. Once seizures are characterized and localized, a risk assessment is performed to weigh the potential of seizure freedom against clinically significant deficits. This requires an informed seizure-onset hypothesis with input from anatomic, electrophysiologic, functional, and neuropsychologic data. Therefore, a multidisciplinary approach is mandatory, involving neurologists, neurosurgeons, neuroradiologists, and neuropsychologists.

The eventual intervention counseling is shared between the patient's neurologist and neurosurgeon. Communication between the neurologist and neurosurgeon must ensure consistent messaging with the patient. The neurologist counsels on the surgical option or options deemed appropriate and expected rates of seizure freedom or, if appropriate, palliation as well as the types of deficits and chances of their occurrence. The neurosurgeon is instrumental in

counseling on the performance of any offered procedure, limitations after surgery, expected recovery, and discussion of potential deficits. It is important to remember that surgery does not need to be completely without risk to be performed, only likely beneficial enough to outweigh the risks involved based on the anticipated change to the quality of life that surgery may provide. The patient ultimately determines this through an informed discussion of the risks and benefits.

Presurgical counseling from the neurologist is also essential to set expectations for postoperative antiseizure medication (ASM) management. Many patients undergo surgical evaluations with the goal of not just seizure freedom but also freedom from ASMs. Neurologist counseling ahead of surgery, and ideally at the start of the surgical evaluation, should be clear that the goal of any surgical intervention is to benefit seizure control but not necessarily eliminate medications. Patients on multiple medications often can reduce doses and eliminate some ASMs over time following successful epilepsy surgery[40,41] but complete ASM removal is not a specific treatment aim.[42]

Immediately following surgery, the neurologist provides inpatient support for any necessary medical management. The neurologist also provides longitudinal follow-up with the timing based on the patient's epilepsy and potential needs. Although timing is not standardized, it is common to perform postoperative EEG over the months and years following surgery to help guide management and assist in prognosis, although data on its utility is mixed.[43,44] Postoperative neuropsychology testing should also be performed within the first 6 to 12 months after surgery to document any new "baseline" cognitive changes compared with preoperative functioning. The decision to reduce or stop ASMs over time can be made at the neurologist's and patient's discretion based on shared decision-making. Early versus late reductions may not alter the overall likelihood of seizure freedom but earlier recurrence may be more likely with earlier reductions.[40]

Neuroradiology Considerations

Neuroradiology plays a central role in the preoperative, operative, and follow-up phases of care for patients undergoing LITT. Preoperative imaging generally consists of standard seizure protocol MRI examinations and potentially single-photon emission computerized tomography (SPECT). An MRI examination should include volumetric images with high spatial resolution and sequences tailored to assess subtle findings. The primary purpose of the initial examination is diagnostic, which should include contrast. High-resolution sequences highlighting gray-white differentiation, such as double inversion recovery or edge enhancing gradient echo, help detect subtle malformations of cortical developement (MCDs) that may not be identifiable on other sequences. However, it may also be used for fusion with subsequent nuclear medicine examinations or neurosurgical procedural planning.

Scrutiny of images for subtle abnormalities such as peri-insular MCDs, subtle MTS, dual pathologic condition, and temporal lobe encephaloceles is critical. When these become available, some findings are only confidently detectable on rereview in the context of nuclear medicine, semiology, and electrophysiologic data.

Additional advanced imaging may be useful for select cases, such as 7 Tesla imaging, diffusion tensor imaging (DTI) with tractography, fluorodeoxyglucose (FDG)-positron emission tomography (PET))/MRI, or functional MRI (fMRI). For example, delineation of the white matter tracts near the insula, such as the arcuate fasciculus with tractography for a left-sided (language dominant) peri-insular ablation planning (**Fig. 3** Insula). The neurosurgeon should be aware that the depicted results of advanced functional imaging methods such as fMRI and DTI with tractography depend on numerous technical and user-dependent parameters. The precise depicted border of white matter tract streamlines, or BOLD activity cannot be assumed to be discrete ground-truth borders. False negatives and false positives occur in all such advanced or mechanistic MRI techniques. This distinction is critical in LITT, as opposed to open, awake craniotomy, where extensive intraoperative mapping can be performed to validate fMRI and tractography findings further. A low threshold for in-person discussion with the neuroradiologist is prudent.

Intraoperative imaging requires stereotactic planning, ablation monitoring, and immediate postablation assessment. Stereotactic images with contrast (MRI or computerized tomography [CT]) are used to plan the trajectories and predicted ablation regions. Routes are selected to avoid blood vessels or preexisting postoperative material and minimize the traversal of sulci and ventricles. There are several additional case-specific or pathology-specific considerations. For example, it is useful to review any advanced imaging performed, such as tractography for trajectories or target areas near eloquent areas; if this is unavailable, detailed knowledge of the expected location of key functional areas of the cerebral cortex as well as white matter tracts on high-resolution anatomic imaging is invaluable.[45] For cavernous malformations, delineating of any associated developmental venous anomalies is useful. For sEEG+/MRI cases, the correlation of planned targets to sEEG lead positions and implicated contacts is vital.

Once the laser fiber(s) are placed, intraoperative MRI is required to confirm fiber position and exclude significant hematoma. The planes and sequences used to monitor ablation are optimized to sequentially depict each fiber's extent of ablation and vulnerable anatomy. During the laser activation for each trajectory, MR thermometry allows near real-time assessment of tissue temperature and an estimated ablation zone with thermal damage threshold lines. One can monitor in 1 to 3 planes; however, as more planes are added, the update time makes the monitoring less "real-time." Low-temperature limits are placed on vulnerable anatomy (eg, 43°C–48°C), and high-temperature limits (eg, 90°C) are set near the laser fiber diffusing tip to surveil for excessive heating or

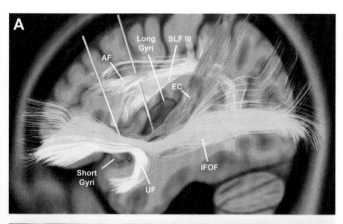

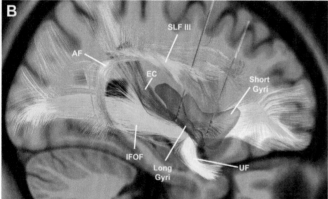

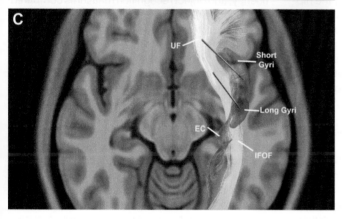

Fig. 3. *Insula: T1-weighted sagittal images with MR tractography demonstrating the relevant tract anatomy for LITT ablation of the insula.* Sagittal T1-weighted imaging from the (*A*) lateral and (*B*) medial projections shows the relationship of the long (red) and short (blue) gyri with the arcuate fasciculus (AF; light orange), superior longitudinal fasciculus part III (SLF III; green), extreme capsule (EC; purple), inferior fronto-occipital fasciculus (IFOF; (cyan). and uncinate fasciculus (UF; yellow). The UF and IFOF traverse the ventral aspect of the claustrum and EC. (*C*) Axial projection with AF and SLF III removed showing the relationship of UF, EC, and IFOF with the insula.

catheter fracture. Commonly protected structures such as the optic tracts or lateral geniculate nucleus can be more difficult to visualize directly on intraoperative imaging, requiring firm knowledge of cross-sectional anatomy to identify confidently. The treating surgeon must constantly visually monitor the heating during each laser ablation to surveil for vapor events should the heating increase more than 100°C. The laser should be immediately turned off. Because PRFS MR thermometry is gradient echo-based, it is important to recognize causes of susceptibility artifacts that may degrade the thermometry, such as blood products (commonly postbiopsy or cavernous malformation) or proximity of the skull base. Lesions that are superficial in the brain may be difficult to evaluate with MR thermometry during LITT if an artifact from a titanium skull anchor bolt is near.

Immediate postprocedure diagnostic imaging with the laser fiber(s) in place helps assess the extent of ablation. Multiple zones of the ablated region have been described. The primary consideration is whether the edge of ablation adequately addresses the lesion or target anatomy for disconnection. This edge is seen as rim enhancement on postgadolinium T1-weighted imaging, T2-weighted FLAIR hyperintensity, and a rim of restricted diffusion surrounding a necrotic core with facilitated diffusion. Recent postablation imaging analyses have suggested that the patients with increased apparent diffusion coefficient (ADC) intensity values on postablation imaging have improved seizure reduction rates after mesial temporal LITT.

The exact evolution of imaging findings over time can vary. Generally, peri-lesional edema increases with a peak around 1 to 3 days and can persist for weeks.[46] Peripheral enhancement persists for months with eventual involution. The volume of ablation can temporarily increase after ablation of focal lesions with subsequent involution and resolution of enhancement, although this is better described for the treatment of neoplasms.[47] One systematic review found that the size of cavernous malformations decreased by 59% on average.[48] Follow-up may also be useful to monitor for recurrence or new lesions when applicable. Downstream effects of network disruption may also indicate successful ablation in some applications, such as a greater decrease in ipsilateral mammillary body size after ablation of the hippocampus in patients with seizure freedom.[22] DTI and tractography might also be useful to directly assess such connectivity changes, although limited data are currently available.[49] In a small series where 4 patients had DTI performed before and after completion of callosotomy, crossing fibers persisted on postop day diffusion imaging in 3 of 4 despite intraoperative imaging demonstrating contrast extravasation in the intended region of the residual corpus callosum. In one patient, no crossing fibers were predicted on postop day one imaging but was detectable on follow-up imaging. Thus, the relationship between the region of LITT lesioning as predicted by intraoperative contrast enhancement and subsequent disconnection gauged by DTI still needs to be fully understood, and further research will be required to identify imaging sequences ideal for the prediction of durable functional disconnection.

A special-case consideration is planning and performing a case in the setting of an implanted medical device such as responsive Neurostimulation (RNS) or vagal nerve stimulation (VNS). Consultation with the radiology MRI safety team, including medical physicists, is imperative. The team can help determine if the procedure can be safely performed (typically at 1.5 Tesla) with a device in place or pulled back or if device removal

would be needed. Additionally, tests can be performed to predict the likely extent and degree of resultant artifact in the areas of interest. This process also helps guide appropriate informed consent. Limited reports of LITT in the setting of implanted devices are available.[50]

Neuropsychology considerations

Neuropsychological assessment is an important component of a comprehensive presurgical epilepsy evaluation. Current recommendations for neuropsychological assessment include administering objective and subjective measures of cognition, emotional, psychosocial, and adaptive functioning.[51] The neuropsychological evaluation provides a cognitive baseline, can help lateralize and localize various cognitive functions, and inform the risk of proposed surgical intervention. In addition, neuropsychological assessment can identify any health-related concerns or psychiatric comorbidities that may need to be addressed preoperatively and/or postoperatively because untreated symptoms of depression and anxiety can influence the quality of life independent of seizure control.[52]

From a cognitive perspective, LITT offers a promising alternative to traditional open resection, such as ATL. Early studies suggest that LITT is associated with fewer postoperative deficits in naming, verbal fluency, and object recognition measures compared with open resection.[12,23] Although there is still the risk of verbal memory decline with LITT in the dominant temporal lobe, there is some evidence of improved memory outcomes. However, research is still ongoing, and further studies with larger samples are needed.[23,53] One critical consideration for surgical planning is whether there are structural abnormalities on neuroimaging because an earlier case study suggests patients with MRI-negative epilepsy may be more likely to experience memory decline following LITT, although this was not replicated in another independent sample.[21,54] Interestingly, a recent study by Kanner and colleagues[55] demonstrated that some patients with preexisting mood and anxiety disorders had improved symptoms following LITT. Furthermore, those with reduced anxiety and depression postoperatively achieved better seizure control. Additionally, in 2 patients with refractory posttraumatic MTLE and posttraumatic stress disorder (PTSD), the amygdala in the ablation zone reduced PTSD-associated psychiatric symptoms, suggesting that tailoring LITT targeting may have the ability to reduce seizures as well as ameliorate common comorbidities (REF 32259241). These studies provide early but encouraging evidence that LITT offers an alternative to open resection that may reduce cognitive morbidity and improve functional outcomes.

Whether patients pursue LITT or open resection, it is critical to consider individual patient characteristics during surgical planning and counseling. No procedure is entirely without risk, and patients have varying risk aversions. It is particularly important to consider each patient's cognitive abilities and level of functioning during the shared decision-making process because previous study shows that those with higher baseline functioning are more likely to experience a decline.[56] Finally, postoperative monitoring is necessary to identify any decline or changes in functional status to facilitate appropriate referrals for additional treatment, such as cognitive rehabilitation or psychotherapy.[51]

SUMMARY

Other forms of thermal ablation are beginning to be used more frequently, such as radiofrequency (RF) and MR-guided ultrasound. However, LITT in epilepsy is by far the most used of these in the United States. Europe, however, has had success historically with RF ablation, and currently, LITT is becoming more popular in areas outside the United States. Because LITT ablations are "tailored" resections that are markedly smaller than what typically occurs in open resections, their seizure freedom rates currently tend to be 10% to 20% less than standard open procedures. From a patient perspective, therapies such as LITT with significantly lower side effect profiles, despite their comparably modest seizure reduction, may render comparable larger improvements in quality from seizure reduction because these gains are not tempered by the quality of life debits from treatment-associated morbidities.[57] However, this is matched by reduced side effects from surgery and fewer complications, which is invaluable to the individual patient. As we improve the targeting of LITT by further studying our interventions at this time and developing ways to improve our tailored techniques with LITT, we hope to find an excellent balance eliminating of seizures with fewer overall complications.

CLINICS CARE POINTS

- *LITT has a prominent role in* MTLE *as a minimally invasive effective technique that may improve patient verbal memory outcomes compared to open selective approaches.*
- LITT has an emerging role in corpus callosotomy; however, long-term efficacy has not been proven.

DISCLOSURES

J.J. Van Gompel M.D: named inventor for intellectual property licensed to Cadence Neuroscience Inc, which is coowned by Mayo Clinic; Investigator for the Medtronic EPAS trial, SLATE trial, and Mayo Clinic Medtronic NIH Public Private Partnership (UH3-NS95495), also with consulting contract; Stock Ownership and Consulting Contract with Neuro-One Inc.; site Primary Investigator in the Polyganics ENCASE II trial; Site Primary Investigator in the NXDC Gleolan Men301 trial; Site Primary Investigator in the Insightec MRgUS EP001 trail. *E.H. Middlebrooks MD:* consultant for Boston Scientific Corp. and Varian Medical Systems, Inc.; receives research funding from Varian Medical Systems. and Vigil Neuroscience, Inc. *D.B. Burkholder MD*; *J.J. Parker MD, PhD*; *S.S. Grewal MD*; *V.T. Lehman MD*; *K.J. Miller MD, PhD*; *E.C. Alden PhD*; and *T.J. Kaufmann MD, MS.*

REFERENCES

1. Blackwell J, Krasny MJ, O'Brien A, et al. Proton resonance frequency shift thermometry: a review of modern clinical practices. J Magn Reson Imaging 2022;55(2):389–403.
2. Penfield W, Flanigin H. The surgical therapy of temporal lobe seizures. Trans Am Neurol Assoc 1950; 51:146–9.
3. Josephson CB, Dykeman J, Fiest KM, et al. Systematic review and meta-analysis of standard vs selective temporal lobe epilepsy surgery. Neurology 2013;80(18):1669–76.
4. Helmstaedter C. Temporal lobe resection–does the prospect of seizure freedom outweigh the cognitive risks? Nat Clin Pract Neurol 2008;4(2): 66–7.
5. Drane DL, Ojemann GA, Aylward E, et al. Category-specific naming and recognition deficits in temporal lobe epilepsy surgical patients. Neuropsychologia 2008;46(5):1242–55.
6. Gastaut H, Gastaut J, Silva GE, et al. Relative frequency of different types of epilepsy: a study employing the classification of the International League Against Epilepsy. Epilepsia 1975;16(3): 457–61.
7. Labate A, Ventura P, Gambardella A, et al. MRI evidence of mesial temporal sclerosis in sporadic "benign" temporal lobe epilepsy. Neurology 2006; 66(4):562–5.
8. Kim WJ, Park SC, Lee SJ, et al. The prognosis for control of seizures with medications in patients with MRI evidence for mesial temporal sclerosis. Epilepsia 1999;40(3):290–3.
9. Kurita T, Sakurai K, Takeda Y, et al. Very long-term outcome of non-surgically treated patients with

temporal lobe epilepsy with hippocampal sclerosis: a retrospective study. PloS one 2016;11(7): e0159464.

10. Picot MC, Baldy-Moulinier M, Daurès JP, et al. The prevalence of epilepsy and pharmacoresistant epilepsy in adults: a population-based study in a Western European country. Epilepsia 2008;49(7):1230–8.

11. Gross RE, Willie JT, Drane DL. The role of stereotactic laser amygdalohippocampotomy in mesial temporal lobe epilepsy. Neurosurg Clin N Am 2016; 27(1):37–50.

12. Drane DL, Loring DW, Voets NL, et al. Better object recognition and naming outcome with MRI-guided stereotactic laser amygdalohippocampotomy for temporal lobe epilepsy. Epilepsia 2015;56(1): 101–13.

13. Jermakowicz WJ, Kanner AM, Sur S, et al. Laser thermal ablation for mesiotemporal epilepsy: analysis of ablation volumes and trajectories. Epilepsia 2017;58(5):801–10.

14. Kang JY, Wu C, Tracy J, et al. Laser interstitial thermal therapy for medically intractable mesial temporal lobe epilepsy. Epilepsia 2016;57(2): 325–34.

15. Waseem H, Osborn KE, Schoenberg MR, et al. Laser ablation therapy: An alternative treatment for medically resistant mesial temporal lobe epilepsy after age 50. Epilepsy Behav : E&B 2015;51:152–7.

16. Petito GT, Wharen RE, Feyissa AM, et al. The impact of stereotactic laser ablation at a typical epilepsy center. Epilepsy Behav 2018;78:37–44.

17. Xue F, Chen T, Sun H. Postoperative outcomes of magnetic resonance imaging (mri)-guided laser interstitial thermal therapy (LITT) in the treatment of drug-resistant epilepsy: a meta-analysis. Med Sci Monit 2018;24:9292–9.

18. Tatum WO, Thottempudi N, Gupta V, et al. De novo temporal intermittent rhythmic delta activity after laser interstitial thermal therapy for mesial temporal lobe epilepsy predicts poor seizure outcome. Clin Neurophysiol 2019;130(1):122–7.

19. Le S, Ho AL, Fisher RS, et al. Laser interstitial thermal therapy (LITT): seizure outcomes for refractory mesial temporal lobe epilepsy. Epilepsy Behav 2018;89:37–41.

20. Grewal SS, Zimmerman RS, Worrell G, et al. Laser ablation for mesial temporal epilepsy: a multi-site, single institutional series. J Neurosurg 2018;1–8. https://doi.org/10.3171/2018.2.JNS171873.

21. Donos C, Breier J, Friedman E, et al. Laser ablation for mesial temporal lobe epilepsy: surgical and cognitive outcomes with and without mesial temporal sclerosis. Epilepsia 2018;59(7):1421–32.

22. Grewal SS, Gupta V, Vibhute P, et al. Mammillary body changes and seizure outcome after laser interstitial thermal therapy of the mesial temporal lobe. Epilepsy Res 2018;141:19–22.

23. Drane DL. MRI-Guided stereotactic laser ablation for epilepsy surgery: promising preliminary results for cognitive outcome. Epilepsy Res 2018;142:170–5.

24. Jermakowicz WJ, Ivan ME, Cajigas I, et al. Visual deficit from laser interstitial thermal therapy for temporal lobe epilepsy: anatomical considerations. Oper Neurosurg (Hagerstown) 2017;13(5):627–33.

25. Wu C, Jermakowicz WJ, Chakravorti S, et al. Effects of surgical targeting in laser interstitial thermal therapy for mesial temporal lobe epilepsy: A multicenter study of 234 patients. Epilepsia 2019;60(6): 1171–83.

26. Téllez-Zenteno JF, Hernández Ronquillo L, Moien-Afshari F, et al. Surgical outcomes in lesional and non-lesional epilepsy: a systematic review and meta-analysis. Epilepsy Res 2010;89(2–3):310–8.

27. Gross RE, Stern MA, Willie JT, et al. Stereotactic laser amygdalohippocampotomy for mesial temporal lobe epilepsy. Ann Neurol 2018;83(3):575–87.

28. Tao JX, Wu S, Lacy M, et al. Stereotactic EEG-guided laser interstitial thermal therapy for mesial temporal lobe epilepsy. J Neurol Neurosurg Psychiatr 2018;89(5):542–8.

29. Youngerman BE, Oh JY, Anbarasan D, et al. Laser ablation is effective for temporal lobe epilepsy with and without mesial temporal sclerosis if hippocampal seizure onsets are localized by stereoelectroencephalography. Epilepsia 2018;59(3):595–606.

30. Sone D, Ahmad M, Thompson PJ, et al. Optimal surgical extent for memory and seizure outcome in temporal lobe epilepsy. Ann Neurol 2022;91(1):131–44.

31. Gupta K, Cabaniss B, Kheder A, et al. Stereotactic MRI-guided laser interstitial thermal therapy for extratemporal lobe epilepsy. Epilepsia 2020;61(8): 1723–34.

32. Perry MS, Donahue DJ, Malik SI, et al. Magnetic resonance imaging-guided laser interstitial thermal therapy as treatment for intractable insular epilepsy in children. J Neurosurg Pediatr 2017;20(6):575–82.

33. Gireesh ED, Lee K, Skinner H, et al. Intracranial EEG and laser interstitial thermal therapy in MRI-negative insular and/or cingulate epilepsy: case series. J Neurosurg 2020;1–9. https://doi.org/10.3171/2020.7.Jns201912.

34. Graham D, Tisdall MM, Gill D. Corpus callosotomy outcomes in pediatric patients: a systematic review. Epilepsia 2016;57(7):1053–68.

35. Jea A, Vachhrajani S, Widjaja E, et al. Corpus callosotomy in children and the disconnection syndromes: a review. Childs Nerv Syst 2008;24(6):685–92.

36. Oguni H, Olivier A, Andermann F, et al. Anterior callosotomy in the treatment of medically intractable epilepsies: a study of 43 patients with a mean follow-up of 39 months. Ann Neurol 1991;30(3): 357–64.

37. Paglioli E, Martins WA, Azambuja N, et al. Selective posterior callosotomy for drop attacks: a new

approach sparing prefrontal connectivity. Neurology 2016;87(19):1968–74.

38. Miller KJ, Fine AL. Decision-making in stereotactic epilepsy surgery. Epilepsia 2022. https://doi.org/10.1111/epi.17381.

39. Ho AL, Miller KJ, Cartmell S, et al. Stereotactic laser ablation of the splenium for intractable epilepsy. Epilepsy Behav Case Rep 2016;5:23–6.

40. Yardi R, Irwin A, Kayyali H, et al. Reducing versus stopping antiepileptic medications after temporal lobe surgery. Ann Clin Transl Neurol 2014;1(2):115–23.

41. Lamberink HJ, Otte WM, Blümcke I, et al. Seizure outcome and use of antiepileptic drugs after epilepsy surgery according to histopathological diagnosis: a retrospective multicentre cohort study. Lancet Neurol 2020;19(9):748–57.

42. Parker JJ, Zhang Y, Fatemi P, et al. Antiseizure medication use and medical resource utilization after resective epilepsy surgery in children in the United States: a contemporary nationwide cross-sectional cohort analysis. Epilepsia 2022;63(4):824–35.

43. Hodges S, Goldenholz DM, Sato S, et al. Postoperative EEG association with seizure recurrence: analysis of the NIH epilepsy surgery database. Epilepsia Open 2018;3(1):109–12.

44. Rathore C, Wattamwar PR, Baheti N, et al. Optimal timing and differential significance of postoperative awake and sleep EEG to predict seizure outcome after temporal lobectomy. Clin Neurophysiol 2018;129(9):1907–12.

45. Kaufmann TJ, Lehman VT, Wong-Kisiel LC, et al. The utility of diffusion tractography for speech preservation in laser ablation of the dominant insula: illustrative case. J Neurosurg Case Lessons 2021;1(19):Case21113.

46. Schwabe B, Kahn T, Harth T, et al. Laser-induced thermal lesions in the human brain: short- and long-term appearance on MRI. J Comput Assist Tomogr 1997;21(5):818–25.

47. Alattar AA, Bartek J Jr, Chiang VL, et al. Stereotactic laser ablation as treatment of brain metastases recurring after stereotactic radiosurgery: a systematic literature review. World Neurosurg 2019;128:134–42.

48. Yousefi O, Sabahi M, Malcolm J, et al. Laser interstitial thermal therapy for cavernous malformations: a systematic review. Front Surg 2022;9:887329.

49. Huang Y, Yecies D, Bruckert L, et al. Stereotactic laser ablation for completion corpus callosotomy. J Neurosurg Pediatr 2019;1–9. https://doi.org/10.3171/2019.5.Peds19117.

50. Buch VP, Mirro EA, Purger DA, et al. Magnetic resonance imaging-guided laser interstitial thermal therapy for refractory focal epilepsy in a patient with a fully implanted RNS system: illustrative case. J Neurosurg Case Lessons 2022;3(21):Case22117.

51. Baxendale S, Wilson SJ, Baker GA, et al. Indications and expectations for neuropsychological assessment in epilepsy surgery in children and adults: Executive summary of the report of the ILAE Neuropsychology Task Force Diagnostic Methods Commission: 2017-2021. Epilepsia 2019;60(9):1794–6.

52. Hamid H, Blackmon K, Cong X, et al. Mood, anxiety, and incomplete seizure control affect quality of life after epilepsy surgery. Neurology 2014;82(10):887–94.

53. Gross RE, Mahmoudi B, Riley JP. Less is more: novel less-invasive surgical techniques for mesial temporal lobe epilepsy that minimize cognitive impairment. Curr Opin Neurol 2015;28(2):182–91.

54. Dredla BK, Lucas JA, Wharen RE, et al. Neurocognitive outcome following stereotactic laser ablation in two patients with MRI-/PET+ mTLE. Epilepsy Behav 2016;56:44–7.

55. Kanner AM, Irving LT, Cajigas I, et al. Long-term seizure and psychiatric outcomes following laser ablation of mesial temporal structures. Epilepsia 2022;63(4):812–23.

56. Helmstaedter C. Cognitive outcomes of different surgical approaches in temporal lobe epilepsy. Epileptic Disord 2013;15(3):221–39.

57. Mahajan UV, Parker JJ, Williams NR, et al. Adjunctive repetitive transcranial magnetic stimulation delivers superior quality of life for focal epilepsy compared to anti-epileptic drugs: a meta-analytic utility prediction study. Brain Stimul 2020;13(2):430–2.

Learning Curve Analysis and Adverse Events After Implementation of Neurosurgical Laser Ablation Treatment
A Population-Based Single-Institution Consecutive Series

Margret Jensdottir, MD[a,b,]*, Ulrika Sandvik, MD, PhD[a,b],
Asgeir S. Jakola, MD, PhD[c,d], Michael Fagerlund, MD, PhD[e],
Annika Kits, MD[e,f], Klara Guðmundsdóttir, MD[a,b], Sara Tabari, MD[a,b],
Tomas Majing, MD[g], Alexander Fletcher-Sandersjöö, MD[a,b],
Clark C. Chen, MD, PhD[h], Jiri Bartek Jr, MD, PhD[a,b,i]

KEYWORDS

- Stereotactic laser ablation • Laser interstitial thermal therapy • Neurosurgery • Complications
- Landriel–Ibanez classification • Learning curve

KEY POINTS

- In this consecutive, single-institution series of the initial 30 patients treated with stereotactic laser ablation (SLA) we show that SLA is a minimally invasive procedure with few adverse events.
- Our results show an improvement of precision of the laser catheter placement and lesion coverage over time indicating a learning curve.
- Four patients (13.3%) experienced new neurological deficits, whereas only one patient had permanent neurological deficits.

INTRODUCTION

Stereotactic laser ablation (SLA), also known as laser interstitial thermal therapy (LITT), is a minimally invasive modality for the treatment of patients with a variety of intracranial lesions, such as brain tumors, radiation necrosis, cavernomas, and epileptogenic foci. It has been used in the United States since 2009[1] and has become increasingly popular to treat deep seated and

a Department of Clinical Neuroscience, Section for Neurosurgery, Karolinska Institutet, Stockholm, Sweden;
b Department of Neurosurgery, Karolinska University Hospital, Hotellet Plan 4, 171 76 Stockholm, Sweden;
c Department of Clinical Neuroscience, Institute of Neuroscience and Physiology, Sahlgrenska Academy, Gothenburg, Sweden; d Department of Neurosurgery, Sahlgrenska University Hospital, Blå stråket 7, plan 3, Sahlgrenska Universitetssjukhuset, 41345 Gothenburg, Sweden; e Department of Neuroradiology, Karolinska University Hospital, ME Neuroradiologi, 171 76 Stockholm, Sweden; f Department of Clinical Neuroscience, Karolinska Institutet; g Funktionsenhet Neuro Operation, Perioperativ Medicin och Intensivvård (PMI), Karolinska Universitetssjukhuset Solna, 171 76 Stockholm Sweden; h Department Chair, Neurosurgery, University of Minnesota Medical School, D429 Mayo Memorial Building, 420 Delaware St. S. E., MMC96, Minneapolis, MN 55455, USA; i Department of Neurosurgery, Rigshospitalet, Copenhagen, Denmark
* Corresponding author. Department of Neurosurgery, Karolinska University Hospital, Hotellet Plan 4, 171 76 Stockholm, Sweden.
E-mail address: margret.jensdottir@regionstockholm.se

Neurosurg Clin N Am 34 (2023) 259–267
https://doi.org/10.1016/j.nec.2022.12.003

previously considered nonsurgically amendable lesions.[2–7]

In anticipation of implementation at our institution, we evaluated the literature to determine the learning curve and opportunities for minimizing adverse events. We studied the current literature describing factors that influence technology adoption in neurosurgery including the ease of adoption if the new technology is built on the foundation of existing technique (ie, SLA based on the concept of stereotaxy).[8] Through this process and in collaboration with the University of Minnesota (UMN), our institution was among the first centers in Europe and the first in the Nordic countries to implement this procedure.[9] Here we present an analysis of our first thirty cases and share our learning curve.

MATERIALS AND METHODS
Study Population Background

The Karolinska University Hospital is a regional referral center serving 2,520,605 inhabitants in 2020 (Source: SCB. Statistics Sweden), with multidisciplinary neuro-oncological care and a multidisciplinary epilepsy surgery team with both adult and pediatric care. All patients were evaluated at a multidisciplinary tumor board for neoplastic lesions or a multidisciplinary epilepsy board.

Laser Ablation Technique

We used the VisualaseTM (Medtronic, Inc, Minneapolis, MN) SLA device, which consists of a laser diode (980 nm wavelength, 15-W), laser fiber, and applicator. The diffusing fiber optic comes in two different lengths of energy output: 3 or 10 mm. A cooling channel allows for circulating sterile saline to assure probe tip cooling. A bone anchor is affixed through a 3.2 mm twist drill hole in the skull to retain the laser applicator along the intended trajectory.

Preoperatively, CT and MR imaging sequences were acquired, and a pretreatment stereotactic planning was performed using Elements stereotaxy (Brainlab) to define the target point for the laser catheter tip, the skull entry point for bone anchor fixation, and an estimate of lesion coverage. The SLA was performed under general anesthesia with the placement of the laser catheter in the operating room using the Leksell frame-based stereotactic system (Elekta AB, Stockholm, Sweden) with O-arm® Surgical Imaging (Medtronic Inc) for the localization of the stereotactic frame and intraoperative verification of the catheter placement. The coordinates for the target and entry points were retrieved after imaging and localization of the stereotactic frame. When the trajectory had

been verified and the laser catheter fixed in place the Leksell arc and the frame was removed, and the patient was transported to the diagnostic MRI suite. A 16-channel flex coil was positioned around the patient's head for imaging acquisition. The MRI (Optima 450w, GE, 1,5 T) was connected to the Visualase console. Imaging planes were selected for continuous thermometry with real-time monitoring of temperature changes during treatment. With the cooling catheter primed and water running a low energy test dose (15% to 25%) was delivered to confirm heat distribution in the intended area. The energy was then increased for the ablation to 45% to 90%. The tissue temperature changes were visualized by the Tmap sequence, and the lesion damage estimate was calculated by the Visualase system and monitored continuously. Ablation was repeated until adequate cell damage had been achieved or had to be stopped due to vicinity of eloquent areas of the brain. If needed, the catheter could be adjusted along the trajectory to ensure optimal ablation.

Postoperatively the patient was in a recovery unit for 2 to 4 h before transfer to the neurosurgical ward and discharged after 24 h observation with corticosteroid tapering over the course of 2 weeks. We routinely used betamethason in a dose of 8 mg twice daily at the day of treatment. The dose was tapered by 2 mg every second day until stopped.

Study Variables

Data were retrospectively assessed including the medical history, patient comorbidities, and neurological examination pre- and postoperatively as well as outcome data. These encompassed patient age, sex, Karnofsky Performance Scale (KPS), treatment indication, prior treatment, clinical presenting symptoms, radiographic data, duration of surgery and hospital stay, histopathology, postoperative neurological deficits, and adverse events within 30 days classified using the Landriel–Ibanez System (**Table 1**).[10] The classification system grades complications according to severity, where grade I is any non-life-threatening event not expected from normal postoperative course, grade II is any complication requiring intervention or treatment, grade III is any life-threatening complication requiring treatment in an intensive care unit, and grade IV is an adverse event leading to death. The grades are further divided into a and b referring to surgical or medical complications respectively. Furthermore, there is a simple correlation between the severity of the adverse events and their grading where Grade I complications are considered mild complications, and Grade II and III complications

Table 1
The Landriel–Ibanez scale of adverse events

Grade I	Any non-life-threatening deviation from normal postoperative course, not requiring invasive treatment
Grade Ia	Complication requiring no drug treatment
Grade Ib	Complication requiring drug treatment
Grade II	Complication requiring invasive treatment such as endovascular interventions
Grade IIa	Complication requiring intervention without general anesthesia
Grade IIb	Complication requiring intervention with general anesthesia
Grade III	Life-threatening complications requiring management in ICU
Grade IIIa	Complication involving single-organ failure
Grade IIIb	Complication involving multiple-organ failure
Grade IV	Complication resulting in death
Surgical complications	Adverse events that are directly related to surgery or surgical technique
Medical complications	Adverse events that are not directly related to surgery or surgical technique

Abbreviation: ICU, intensive care unit.
From Landriel Ibanez FA, Hem S, Ajler P, Vecchi E, Ciraolo C, Baccanelli M, Tramontano R, Knezevich F, Carrizo A (2011) A new classification of complications in neurosurgery. World Neurosurg 75:709-715; discussion 604-711.

are considered moderate and severe, respectively. Complications were further subdivided into technical complications or hyperthermia-related complications.

The Elements stereotaxy software (Brainlab®, Munich Germany) was used to measure and calculate the accuracy of data. The accuracy of the target and entry point was measured as the 2D radial distance in mm between the catheter tip and the planned target point and the skull entry point and the planned entry point, respectively. Pre- and posttreatment tumor and ablation volumes (MRI contrast-enhanced T1) were also determined using the Brainlab elements software (Brainlab®, Munich Germany) segmentation tool.

The ablation volume was defined as the total volume of thermally induced irreversible cell damage within a margin of a thin enhancing rim (peripheral enhancing rim), seen in the post-ablation MRI. A definition previously described in detail.[11–13]

Statistics

Data are presented as median (interquartile range) or number (proportion). To identify learning curves, we generated scatterplots and calculated the Pearson correlation coefficient (PCC) between the cumulative number of procedures performed and clinically important outcome measures (OR time, lesion coverage, target point (TP)-deviation, entry point (EP)-deviation, and frame deviation). In short, PCC measures the linear correlation between X and Y and generates a correlation coefficient ("R") from -1 to 1, where 1 implies a perfect linear relationship, -1 suggests a perfect inverse linear relationship, and 0 indicates no linear dependency. We chose to use PCC, as opposed to, for example, Spearman or Kendall correlation, as all of the outcome measures were parametric or near-parametric, and both the outcome and explanatory values are measured on the continuous scale. All analyses were conducted using the statistical software program R (version 4.1.2), and statistical significance was set at $P < .05$.

Ethics and Approvals

The Regional Committee for Medical and Health Research Ethics in Stockholm approved the study protocol and waived the need for signed consent (Dnr: 2017/1760–31/1).

RESULTS
Baseline Data

Thirty patients were included. Clinical, radiographic, and treatment data are shown in **Tables 2–4**. Patients were treated for either a recurrent glioma (57%), de novo glioma (23%), or an epileptic foci (20%). The median time from diagnosis to surgery was 35 days, and the median OR time was 252 min. The median lesion volume was 1.2 cm^3, and 60% of patients had a lesion coverage of 100% (IQR 90% to 100%).

Learning Curve

Scatterplots between the cumulative number of procedures performed and clinically important outcome measures are presented in **Fig. 1**. With an increasing number of cases there was significant decrease in EP-deviation ($R = -0.39$, $P = .034$), and a near-significant decrease in TP-deviation

Table 2
Baseline characteristics

Variable	All Patients (n = 30)
Female sex	12 (40%)
Age (y)	48 (33 to 56)
Karnofsky Performance Status	90 (80 to 90) (4 missing)
Prior tumor resection	17 (57%)
Prior biopsy	8 (27%)
Clinical presentation	
Seizures	18 (60%)
Headaches	1 (3.3%)
Cognitive deficits	3 (10%)
Motor deficits	5 (17%)
Speech deficits	5 (17%)
Visual deficits	4 (13%)
Treatment indication (according to Hawasli et al)[30]	
1: Deep-seated glial neoplasm	7 (23%)
2: Recurrent glioma	17 (57%)
3: Recurrent metastasis post radiosurgery	0 (0%)
4: Deep-seated epilepsy focus	6 (20%)
Diagnostic radiological work-up	
Transcranial magnetic stimulation	4 (13%)
Diffusion tensor imaging	27 (90%)
Functional MRI	8 (27%)
Positron emission tomography	7 (23%)

Data were presented as count (proportion) or median (IQR).

Table 3
Radiological and histopathological characteristics

Variable	All Patients (n = 30)
Lesion location	
Basal ganglia	1 (3.3%)
Frontal	8 (27%)
Frontoparietal	1 (3.3%)
Hypothalamus	1 (3.3%)
Insula	3 (10%)
Occipital	1 (3.3%)
Parietal	1 (3.3%)
Splenium	3 (10%)
Temporal	7 (23%)
Third ventricle	4 (13%)
Lesion side	
Central	6 (20%)
Left	13 (43%)
Right	11 (37%)
Lesion shape	
Asymmetrical	6 (20%)
Ellipsoid	11 (37%)
Spherical	13 (43%)
Lesion volume (cm³)	1.2 (0.5 to 2.9)
Contrast enhancing	25 (83%)
Peritumoral edema	10 (33%)
Eloquent area	12 (40%)
Pathology report	
Astrocytoma grade 2	1 (3.3%)
Astrocytoma grade 3	2 (6.7%)
Cavernoma	3 (10%)
Ependymoma	1 (3.3%)
Focal cortical dysplasia	3 (10%)
Glioblastoma	11 (37%)
Oligodendroglioma grade 2	3 (10%)
Oligodendroglioma grade 3	2 (6.7%)
Pilocytic astrocytoma	4 (13%)

Data were presented as count (proportion) or median (IQR).

($R = -0.34$, $P = .070$). EP- and TP-deviation both stabilized after approximately 15 cases (see **Fig. 1**C, D). With an increasing number of cases, there was also a near-significant increase in lesion coverage ($R = 0.36$, $P = .052$), implying more complete ablation of the target lesion with experience. This association appeared to stabilize after approximately 20 to 25 procedures were performed (see **Fig. 1**B). There were no changes in OR-time (see **Fig. 1**A) or frame accuracy (see **Fig. 1**E, F) with a cumulative number of procedures.

Adverse Events

Hyperthermic complications occurred in three patients and was the result of inadequate irrigation in two of the cases. In a patient treated with two catheters, the irrigation was not connected to the proper laser catheter after switching between the first and the second catheters. During the low energy test dose for the second catheter, we acknowledged this, and the irrigation was properly connected. A small, subclinical, hyperintense lesion occurred on the MRI. In the second patient, there was a technical complication with leakage at

Table 4
Outcome data

Variable	All Patients ($n = 30$)
Time from diagnosis to surgery (d)	35 (15 to 75)
Duration of surgery (min)	252 (229 to 298)
Extent of lesion coverage (%)	100 (90 to 100)
Catheters	
One	26 (87%)
Two	4 (13%)
Accuracy	
Catheter entry point deviation (mm)	0.8 (0.4 to 1.0)
Catheter target point deviation (mm)	0.9 (0.7 to 1.5)
Frame mean deviation (mm)[a]	0.3 (0.2 to 0.3)
Frame max deviation (mm)[a]	0.8 (0.7 to 0.8)
Hospital stay (d)	1.0 (1.0 to 2.0)
Surgical complication	11 (37%)
Hyperthermic complication	3 (10%)
Technical complication	1 (3.3%)
Ibanez grade	
Ibanez grade Ia	5 (17%)
Ibanez grade Ib	3 (10%)
Ibanez grade IIa	2 (6.7%)
Ibanez grade IIb	1 (3.3%)

Data presented as count (proportion) or median (IQR).
Abbreviations: min, minutes; mm, millimeters.
[a] 4 missing values, $n = 26$.

the irrigation connection site, resulting in an inadequate cooling of the laser catheter during a part of the treatment. This was recognized as a hyperintensity in the white matter along the catheter tract on T2/flair imaging (**Fig. 2**). However, no symptoms could be related to this finding. The third patient, treated for a tumor in the third ventricle, suffered from temporary hypothalamic disturbance from day 3 after treatment and was readmitted to the hospital for observation and medical treatment for fluid- and electrolyte disturbance. Although not visible as a lesion on the MRI it was classified as a hyperthermic complication. Ibanez grade II event occurred in 3 patients—all wound infections requiring debridement with either local ($n = 2$) or general anesthesia ($n = 1$). No serious adverse event occurred and there was no procedural-related death or mortality within 30 days.

DISCUSSION

In this consecutive, single-institution series of the initial 30 patients treated with SLA at our institution after the technique has been implemented, we show that SLA is a minimally invasive procedure with few adverse events. Our results show an improvement of precision and lesion coverage over time.

Learning Curve

The success of the laser ablation is dependent on correct placement of the laser catheter, as poor positioning can result in inadequate ablation or adverse events such as hemorrhage or unintended hyperthermia in normal brain tissue.[14] Although the accuracy of the various stereotactic systems is well described.,[3,15–17] how best to adapt these systems to the laser ablation equipment and probe remain unclear. As a first step to address this issue, we measured the deviation of the laser catheter placed using our frame-based stereotaxy workflow from the planned trajectory. We found a median deviation of 0.8 mm and 0.9 mm at the entry and target point, respectively. This corresponds to a very high accuracy. Few studies on SLA have reported accuracy data in a similar manner. Attaar and colleagues[18] reported a mean radial error of 0.9 ± 1.6 mm using a frameless stereotaxy, where 65% of lasers were deemed to be exactly on the planned trajectory. For the 30 procedures that deviated from the planned trajectory they reported a mean radial error of 2.6 ± 1.9 mm. Shofty and colleagues[19] also reported an accuracy of the laser catheter from the planned trajectory in a similar manner as in our study, with errors ranging from 0 to 5.9 mm and abortion of 1 procedure due to laser catheter misplacement. Despite this, they did not experience any intracranial hemorrhage or neurological complications in their cohort.

Although the incidence of laser catheter misplacement in previous studies has been reported at around 2% to 5%,[20–22] we did not have to reposition a laser catheter or abort the procedure due to laser misplacement in any patient. However, we were forced to abort one treatment half-way through due to technical complication with leakage of irrigation fluid in the MRI from the cooling catheter connection. This patient did not experience any clinically relevant adverse event even though this also resulted in a hyperthermic complication, defined by a T2/flair hyperintensity

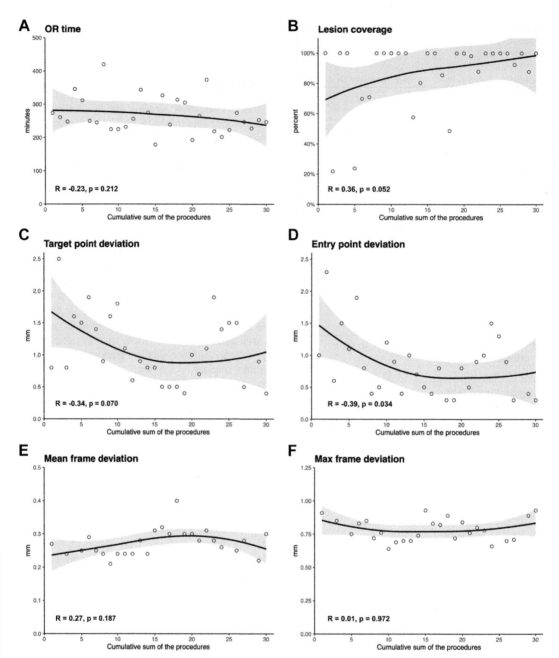

Fig. 1. Pearson correlation coefficients, scatterplots, and LOESS-curves showing the correlation between the cumulative sum of the procedures performed and OR-time (*A*), lesion coverage (*B*), target point deviation (*C*), entry point deviation (*D*), mean frame deviation (*E*), and max frame deviation (*F*).

along the laser catheter due to inadequate cooling for a short period of time.

An indication of a learning curve for the laser catheter placement was observed in our cohort, with a significant association for EP-deviation and a near-significant association for TP-deviation, which stabilized after approximately 15 performed cases. Patel and colleagues[22] reported his experience of 20 patients and a subsequent development of a standardized procedure

protocol that lowered the incidence of hemorrhage, inaccurate laser placement, thermal injury and perioperative death with increasing experience. Similarly, Jethwa and colleagues[21] reported improved accuracy of laser insertion with increased experience. Furthermore, they observed a shift in patient selection, with an average lesion diameter of 2.13 cm for the first 10 patients and 1.65 cm in the following 10 patients, as an indicator of learning curve for SLA—

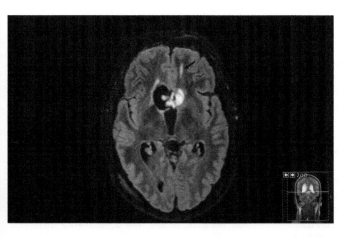

Fig. 2. Axial T2/flair MRI. Hyperthermic complication showed as a hyperintensity in the white matter of the left frontal lobe (*arrow*), following the catheter tract.

that is, the surgeon embracing the limitations of the technique in terms of lesion size.

We also noted a near-significant learning curve of gradually increasing lesion coverage, which stabilized after approximately 20 to 25 procedures performed. This is like what other studies report, with better lesion coverage and ablation volumes with increased experience but also a tendency to select cases with smaller lesions[23] as mentioned above. However, the comparison to previous literature is impeded by several factors, especially the large variety of tumor volumes treated in other series (with a range from 1.2-62.78[24–27]), which could influence the probability of achieving complete ablation.

Finally, although a decrease in operating time with increased experience is a common indicator of a learning curve,[23,28] we did not find any association over time in our cohort.

Adverse Events

In addition to the ability to treat deep-seated lesions, the potential benefits of SLA compared with open surgery are likely related to the minimally invasive nature of the modality with lower risk of serious complications. Nevertheless, in the implementation phase, one might expect a higher rate of adverse events. As there is no literature addressing this, we looked at the more general figures reporting nonnegligible mortality frequency of 2% to 5% 30-day mortality rate[21,23,25,29–32] and adverse events frequency at 13% to 41%[21,23,25,30–32] In the largest reported cohort so far of 238 patients treated with SLA, Shao and colleagues[23] report 30.2% new neurological deficits following treatment. The reported adverse events are nevertheless difficult to interpret as standardization is lacking.

In our cohort, we did not experience any fatalities related to the treatment, although eleven patients experienced some form of adverse event. Four patients (13,3%) suffered from new neurological deficits (1 patient had difficulties with fine motor skills of the right hand, 2 patients experienced temporary speech disturbances and 1 patient had a permanent hemiparesis although improving form initial hemiplegia after treatment). In addition, 3 patients had some signs of surgical site infection, although only 1 patient (3,3%) had to undergo surgical debridement using general anesthesia. We postulate that this might have occurred due to burning of the skin while drilling through a small incision. We have since adapted a meticulous irrigation during drilling to avoid injuring the skin.

Surgical site infection is a known complication that increases the risk of morbidity and mortality. However, this has not been addressed in a systematic manner in the literature, although in SLA there seems to be a reported rate of infection of around 1% to 3%.[31] With respect to postprocedural hemorrhage, literature reports an approx. 3% incidence of significant procedural hemorrhage requiring surgical intervention.[22,23] We had no such cases, with meticulous care taken in the preoperative planning to avoid puncture or ablation too close to large blood vessels.[33] Our results suggest that SLA carries few serious adverse events even in the startup phase of implementation, although lack of similar reports and the lack of standardized reporting of adverse events makes comparing results difficult. We have adopted a more stringent care of the skin during drilling and closure of the wound to try to avoid infection at the surgical site.

Limitations

This is a retrospective study with its inherent limitations, such as the bias of patient selection and only a crude end point concerning effectiveness.

Furthermore, despite using a standardized way of reporting adverse events, one may not reveal the entire spectrum of neurological disabilities and/or complications due to the limitation of the Landriel–Ibanez. A further limitation of this classification system is the definition of a persistent neurological deficit as a deficit extending beyond 30 days of the surgical procedure, whereas a majority of publications report a neurological deficit as persistent when extending beyond 90 days. Although this work does have its limitations, only very few series reporting the initial experience of SLA to exist, and our study group is, to the best of our knowledge, the only one using a standardized classification system. As such, we believe our study can be useful for centers considering implementation of SLA in their practice, who can hopefully benefit and learn from our experience regarding what to expect in the startup phase in terms of learning curve and adverse events.

SUMMARY

Even though there is a learning over the first 30 cases, our results indicate that the technique can safely be implemented at established neurosurgical centers with experience of stereotaxy. Comparison of learning curve and adverse events is hampered by non-standardized reports in the literature and we recommend embracing a more standardized system when it comes to reporting outcomes.

DISCLOSURE

The authors have nothing to disclose.

CLINICS CARE POINTS

- Stereotactic laser ablation is a minimally invasive treatment modality for ablation of neoplastic or epileptic lesions by thermal damage under continuous monitoring with MRI.
- The success of the laser ablation is highly dependent on correct placement of the laser catheter, as poor positioning can result in inadequate ablation or adverse events such as hemorrhage or unintended hyperthermia in normal brain tissue.
- Meticulous care has to be taken in the pre-planning of the laser ablation on recent preoperative MRI.
- The treatment is minimally invasive with usually a short hospital stay (1 to 2 days).

ACKNOWLEDGMENTS

The authors acknowledge the help of NOCRiiC with this research.

REFERENCES

1. Chen C, Lee I, Tatsui C, et al. Laser interstitial thermotherapy (LITT) for the treatment of tumors of the brain and spine: a brief review. J Neurooncol 2021; 151:429–42.
2. Alattar AA, Bartek J Jr, Chiang VL, et al. Stereotactic laser ablation as treatment of brain metastases recurring after stereotactic radiosurgery: a systematic literature review. World Neurosurg 2019;128: 134–42.
3. Ashraf O, Patel NV, Hanft S, et al. Laser-induced thermal therapy in neuro-oncology: a review. World Neurosurg 2018;112:166–77.
4. Carpentier A, McNichols RJ, Stafford RJ, et al. Laser thermal therapy: real-time MRI-guided and computer-controlled procedures for metastatic brain tumors. Lasers Surg Med 2011;43:943–50.
5. Johnson RA, Do TH, Palzer EF, et al. Pattern of technology diffusion in the adoption of stereotactic laser interstitial thermal therapy (LITT) in neuro-oncology. J Neurooncol 2021;153:417–24.
6. North RY, Raskin JS, Curry DJ. MRI-guided laser interstitial thermal therapy for epilepsy. Neurosurg Clin N Am 2017;28:545–57.
7. Zemmar A, Nelson BJ, Neimat JS. Laser thermal therapy for epilepsy surgery: current standing and future perspectives. Int J Hyperthermia 2020;37: 77–83.
8. Wilson CB. Adoption of new surgical technology. BMJ 2006;332:112–4.
9. Bartek J Jr, Kits A, Jensdottir M. Laser ablation of brain tumors now available in the Nordic countries. Lakartidningen 2020;117:19260 [in Swedish].
10. Landriel Ibanez FA, Hem S, Ajler P, et al. A new classification of complications in neurosurgery. World Neurosurg 2011;75:709–15.
11. Kahn T, Bettag M, Ulrich F, et al. MRI-guided laser-induced interstitial thermotherapy of cerebral neoplasms. J Comput Assist Tomogr 1994;18:519–32.
12. Parisi AJ, Sundararajan SH, Garg R, et al. Assessment of optimal imaging protocol sequences after laser-induced thermal therapy for intracranial tumors. Neurosurgery 2018;83:471–9.
13. Salem U, Kumar VA, Madewell JE, et al. Neurosurgical applications of MRI guided laser interstitial thermal therapy (LITT). Cancer Imaging 2019;19:65.
14. Pruitt R, Gamble A, Black K, et al. Complication avoidance in laser interstitial thermal therapy: lessons learned. J Neurosurg 2017;126:1238–45.
15. Bartek J Jr, Alattar A, Jensdottir M, et al. Biopsy and ablation of H3K27 glioma using skull-mounted

smartframe device: technical case report. World Neurosurg 2019;127:436–41.

16. Lagman C, Chung LK, Pelargos PE, et al. Laser neurosurgery: a systematic analysis of magnetic resonance-guided laser interstitial thermal therapies. J Clin Neurosci 2017;36:20–6.

17. Patel NV, Mian M, Stafford RJ, et al. Laser interstitial thermal therapy technology, physics of magnetic resonance imaging thermometry, and technical considerations for proper catheter placement during magnetic resonance imaging-guided laser interstitial thermal therapy. Neurosurgery 2016;79(Suppl 1):S8–16.

18. Attaar SJ, Patel NV, Hargreaves E, et al. Accuracy of laser placement with frameless stereotaxy in magnetic resonance-guided laser-induced thermal therapy. Oper Neurosurg (Hagerstown) 2015;11:554–63.

19. Shofty B, Bergman L, Berger A, et al. Adopting MR-guided stereotactic laser ablations for epileptic lesions: initial clinical experience and lessons learned. Acta Neurochir (Wien) 2021;163:2797–803.

20. Arocho-Quinones EV, Lew SM, Handler MH, et al. Magnetic resonance-guided stereotactic laser ablation therapy for the treatment of pediatric brain tumors: a multiinstitutional retrospective study. J Neurosurg Pediatr 2020;26:13–21.

21. Jethwa PR, Barrese JC, Gowda A, et al. Magnetic resonance thermometry-guided laser-induced thermal therapy for intracranial neoplasms: initial experience. Neurosurgery 2012;71:133–44, 144-135.

22. Patel P, Patel NV, Danish SF. Intracranial MR-guided laser-induced thermal therapy: single-center experience with the Visualase thermal therapy system. J Neurosurg 2016;125:853–60.

23. Shao J, Radakovich NR, Grabowski M, et al. Lessons learned in using laser interstitial thermal therapy for treatment of brain tumors: a case series of 238 patients from a single institution. World Neurosurg 2020;139:e345–54.

24. Hawasli AH, Kim AH, Dunn GP, et al. Stereotactic laser ablation of high-grade gliomas. Neurosurg Focus 2014;37:E1.

25. Mohammadi AM, Sharma M, Beaumont TL, et al. Upfront magnetic resonance imaging-guided stereotactic laser-ablation in newly diagnosed glioblastoma: a multicenter review of survival outcomes compared with a matched cohort of biopsy-only patients. Neurosurgery 2019;85:762–72.

26. Rennert RC, Khan U, Tatter SB, et al. Patterns of clinical use of stereotactic laser ablation: analysis of a multicenter prospective registry. World Neurosurg 2018;116:e566–70.

27. Viozzi I, Guberinic A, Overduin CG, et al. Laser interstitial thermal therapy in patients with newly diagnosed glioblastoma: a systematic review. J Clin Med 2021;10(2):355.

28. Taha BR, Osswald CR, Rabon M, et al. Learning curve associated with clearpoint neuronavigation system: a case series. World Neurosurg X 2022; 13:100115.

29. Dabecco R, Gigliotti MJ, Mao G, et al. Laser interstitial thermal therapy (LITT) for intracranial lesions: a single-institutional series, outcomes, and review of the literature. Br J Neurosurg 2021;1–7. https://doi.org/10.1080/02688697.2021.1947972.

30. Hawasli AH, Bagade S, Shimony JS, et al. Magnetic resonance imaging-guided focused laser interstitial thermal therapy for intracranial lesions: single-institution series. Neurosurgery 2013;73:1007–17.

31. Kamath AA, Friedman DD, Hacker CD, et al. MRI-guided interstitial laser ablation for intracranial lesions: a large single-institution experience of 133 cases. Stereotact Funct Neurosurg 2017;95:417–28.

32. Patel PD, Patel NV, Davidson C, et al. The role of MRgLITT in overcoming the challenges in managing infield recurrence after radiation for brain metastasis. Neurosurgery 2016;79(Suppl 1):S40–58.

33. Rodriguez A, Tatter SB. Laser ablation of recurrent malignant gliomas: current status and future perspective. Neurosurgery 2016;79(Suppl 1):S35–9.

Neurosurgical Applications of Magnetic Hyperthermia Therapy

Daniel Rivera, BS[a,b,c,1], Alexander J. Schupper, MD[a,1],
Alexandros Bouras, MD[b,c], Maria Anastasiadou, PhD[a],
Lawrence Kleinberg, MD[d], Dara L. Kraitchman, VMD, PhD, MS[e],
Anilchandra Attaluri, PhD[f], Robert Ivkov, PhD[d,g,h,i],
Constantinos G. Hadjipanayis, MD, PhD[a,b,c,*]

KEYWORDS

- Magnetic hyperthermia therapy • Magnetic fluid hyperthermia • Glioblastoma
- Magnetic particle imaging • Thermotherapy • Brain neoplasms • High-grade glioma

KEY POINTS

- Magnetic hyperthermia therapy is a highly localized and remotely controllable form of hyperthermia therapy that uses an alternating magnetic field to heat magnetic nanoparticles delivered to the tumor target.
- In addition to causing direct inhibitory and cytotoxic effects on tumor cells, magnetic hyperthermia therapy may enhance the effectiveness of standard radiotherapy and chemotherapy drugs used for high-grade gliomas through multiple mechanisms.
- Magnetic hyperthermia therapy is generally well tolerated and, when combined with radiation therapy, is associated with overall survival benefits in patients with malignant brain tumors; however, significant technical challenges limit its current clinical use in neurosurgery.
- As the nanoparticles may stay in position for weeks to months, multiple sessions of magnetic hyperthermia therapy can be performed over time, allowing for optimization of the timing of heat therapy with relation to radiotherapy and potential enhancement of the therapeutic ratio.
- Incorporating improved magnetic nanoparticle delivery methods, visualization of their distribution in the tissue, and noninvasive real-time thermometry into treatment planning is critical to advancing this treatment modality for patients.

[a] Department of Neurological Surgery, Icahn School of Medicine at Mount Sinai, 1 Gustave L. Levy Place, New York, NY 10029, USA; [b] Department of Neurological Surgery, University of Pittsburgh, 200 Lothrop Street, Suite F-158, Pittsburgh, PA 15213, USA; [c] Brain Tumor Nanotechnology Laboratory, UPMC Hillman Cancer Center, 5117 Centre Avenue, Pittsburgh, PA 15232, USA; [d] Department of Radiation Oncology and Molecular Radiation Sciences, Johns Hopkins University, 1550 Orleans Street, Baltimore, MD 21231-5678, USA; [e] Russell H Morgan Department of Radiology and Radiological Science, Johns Hopkins University, 600 North Wolfe Street, Baltimore, MD 21287, USA; [f] Department of Mechanical Engineering, The Pennsylvania State University, 777 West Harrisburg Pike Middletown, PA 17057, USA; [g] Department of Oncology, Johns Hopkins University School of Medicine, 1550 Orleans Street, Baltimore, MD 21231-5678, USA; [h] Department of Mechanical Engineering, Johns Hopkins University, Whiting School of Engineering, 3400 North Charles Street, Baltimore, MD 21218, USA; [i] Department of Materials Science and Engineering, Johns Hopkins University, Whiting School of Engineering, 3400 North Charles Street, Baltimore, MD 21218, USA
[1] Co-first authorship.
* Corresponding author.
E-mail address: hadjipanayiscg2@upmc.edu

Neurosurg Clin N Am 34 (2023) 269–283
https://doi.org/10.1016/j.nec.2022.11.004

INTRODUCTION TO MAGNETIC HYPERTHERMIA THERAPY

Hyperthermia therapy (HT) is a treatment modality where the temperature of a region of the body or the whole body is elevated above baseline temperatures to treat the disease. Although HT can treat a variety of infections and diseases, the focus over the past half-century is to apply HT to treat various forms of cancer.[1-3] For HT to be effective, the temperature in approximately 90% of the target volume, referred to as T_{90}, must reach the minimum effective thermal dose.[4,5] Heating tumors to temperatures between 40°C and 45°C causes changes that are toxic to both tumor vasculature and the cancer cells themselves.[6-8] These changes include inducing apoptosis and protein damage, activating antitumor immune responses, and initiating vasodilation to enhance intratumoral blood flow that improves drug distribution and chemotherapy (CT) and increases tumor oxygenation for more effective radiation therapy (RT).[4,9-15] Heat-based therapies also transiently increase blood–brain barrier (BBB) and blood–tumor barrier (BTB) permeability, potentially allowing for lower dose CT to achieve therapeutic levels within brain tumors.[16,17] It is important to note that HT is distinct from fever in that HT, even when applied to the whole body, does not alter the hypothalamic temperature set point.[18] Although HT can be applied nonspecifically to the entire body, local hyperthermia produces fewer side effects.[19] Even still, optimal clinical implementation within the central nervous system (CNS) requires developing a practical means to appropriately target the delivery of heat and confirm the extent of temperature elevation with precise thermometry.

Magnetic nanoparticles (MNPs) represent a precision tool to perform highly localized HT known as magnetic hyperthermia therapy (MHT). After local delivery of the MNPs, an external alternating magnetic field (AMF) is applied to heat the MNPs **Fig. 1**. The potential mechanisms through which the MNPs convert the electromagnetic energy produced by the AMF into heat include magnetic hysteresis losses and Brownian relaxation, a process in which heat is generated by the physical rotation of the MNPs.[19,20] For spherical MNPs, the former mechanism dominates. The heating efficiency of MHT is largely determined by the size, shape, and composition of the MNPs, as well as the frequency and field amplitude of the AMF.[21] The specific loss power (SLP), or specific absorption rate (SAR), is a term used to characterize the heating efficiency of MNPs and is defined as the measured thermal loss normalized by mass or volume of magnetic material.[22,23] Though commonly used, SAR in this context is ambiguous and can lead to confusion. Heat absorbed by tissues exposed to electromagnetic fields is defined as SAR by the US Federal Communications Commission (FCC), which regulates electromagnetic radiation sources and their use.[24] Tissues exposed to the AMF during MHT will thus heat from two sources—directly from interactions with the AMF and indirectly from hysteresis heat produced by the MNPs. For clinical applications, we thus recommend the use of SLP when referring to MNP heat generation.

Common materials used to synthesize MNPs include manganese, cobalt, iron, and nickel. However, magnetite (Fe_3O_4) and maghemite (γ-Fe_2O_3) nanoparticles, collectively known as magnetic iron oxide nanoparticles (MIONPs), are the only MNPs approved for human use and have been extensively studied for MHT due to their heating capabilities and established record of biocompatibility and safety.[25-28] In addition to being excellent heating agents, MNPs possess additional therapeutic

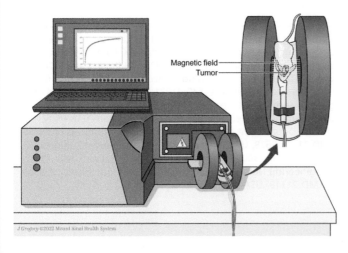

Fig. 1. Illustration of rodent MHT following intracranial MIONP delivery.

Magnetic field
Tumor

J Gregory ©2022 Mount Sinai Health System

and diagnostic capabilities as contrast agents, drug-carriers and chemo-radiosensitizers.[29–37] Although MIONPs have significant therapeutic potential with an established safety record, toxicity is typically related to excessive or rapid iron release which depends on the nanoparticle coating, dose, and mode of administration.[38,39] The metabolic rate of the tissue into which they are deposited also plays a role in MNP-associated toxicity.[40–42] As the effectiveness of MHT is determined by the lowest thermal dose generated within the target region, it is important to design MNPs that generate significant heat at low concentrations to maximize therapeutic efficacy and minimize toxicity.[43]

Despite the non-specific application of the AMF to the body, localized MHT can be achieved by delivering the MNPs specifically to the tumor area, minimizing potentially harmful off-target heating. Local delivery of MNPs occurs either through targeted systemic delivery or direct intratumoral deposition, either by stereotactic injection or a technique known as convection-enhanced delivery (CED).[44–46] Targeted systemic delivery is most often accomplished by conjugating MNPs or MNP-encapsulating vesicles with cancer-specific moieties and administering them intravenously.[47–49] In addition, systemically delivered MNPs may be guided to the region of interest by applying an external static magnetic field to direct MNPs toward the tumor area.[50] Previous studies reported the use of a multi-trajectory installation of multiple MNP depots using neuro-navigation depending on the tumor location and geometry to obtain a more homogenous distribution.[51] CED is currently being studied as a method to deliver MNPs for MHT into the brain, as it bypasses the BBB and minimizes potentially toxic systemic effects.

Advantages of Magnetic Hyperthermia Therapy for the Treatment of Brain Cancer

In 1957, MHT was first explored as a treatment of cancer that had metastasized to the lymph nodes in a canine study.[52] Since then, MHT has been attempted *in vitro* and *in vivo* to treat a variety of cancers, including head and neck, pancreas, lung, prostate, breast, and brain.[4,53–61] In all cases, MHT can increase intratumoral temperatures, promote cancer cell death, and inhibit tumor growth.

In neurosurgery, MHT has been applied mainly to treat aggressive and therapy-resistant forms of brain cancer such as glioblastoma (GBM). As with other high-grade gliomas (HGGs), GBM is characterized by infiltrative growth into healthy surrounding brain tissue, as well as high levels of tumor cell heterogeneity.[62,63] Despite an intense standard of care therapeutic scheme consisting of maximal safe tumor resection followed by fractionated RT and concomitant and adjuvant temozolomide (TMZ) CT, prognosis remains poor for patients with GBM.[64–66] Recent FDA approval of 5-aminolevulinic acid (5-ALA) as an intraoperative imaging agent for fluorescence-guided surgery has significantly increased the average extent of tumor resection. However, due to its infiltrative nature and tendency to invade eloquent regions of the brain, total resection of GBM tumors remains unfeasible despite enhanced intraoperative tumor visualization.[65–72] Infiltrative tumor cells, including GBM stem-like cells (GSCs), that are left behind after tumor resection at the tumor margin and in the surrounding healthy brain often develop therapy resistance and are mediators of the invariable local and lethal recurrence that makes GBM refractory.[62,73,74] Despite decades of research, GBM remains one of the greatest challenges facing neurosurgical oncology due to limitations in drug delivery across the BBB and therapy resistance.[68–70]

Hyperthermia has been shown to enhance the cytotoxicity of RT to tumor cells. Since then, there have been numerous attempts to combine the two therapies and develop a feasible and effective approach in the clinical management of a variety of tumor types including GBM.[75] There are several distinct processes that may contribute to this biologic effect, although the dominant mechanism remains uncertain. HT initiates intracellular heat shock response(s) that disrupt the repair of radiation-induced double-strand DNA breaks.[76–80] HT also degrades or denatures the DNA repair pathway protein BRCA2.[81,82] Moderate HT, which increases perfusion, may also increase radiosensitivity by reducing the radioresistant hypoxic cell populations. More recently, HT has been investigated as a means to disrupt the BBB thereby enhancing drug delivery to brain tumors such that the effectiveness of DNA-damaging systemic drugs, such as TMZ and immune-oncologic agents, is improved.[83–86]

MHT has the potential to be highly relevant to future treatment of HGGs and was approved in Europe in 2012 as an adjuvant therapy for recurrent GBM in combination with RT.[87] In addition to providing all the advantages of HT (ie, opening of the BBB, induction of apoptosis, enhanced antitumor immune response), MHT additionally possesses unique features that overcome many limitations of other heat-based therapies commonly used to treat brain tumors. First, MIONPs radiosensitize GBM cells and induce apoptosis in the GSCs thought to mediate local recurrence.[88,89] In addition, AMF penetration depth exceeds that of other activating modalities used in HT, such as light or acoustic waves.[25] Unlike other thermal therapies such as laser interstitial thermal therapy (LITT) which may only be performed intraoperatively, MHT can be performed after post-operative recovery and the initiation of RT in a minimally invasive manner through the application of an external AMF that reaches deep-seated tumors through skin and bone without incision.[25] Furthermore, MNPs can be administered at the time of surgical resection, sparing the patient an additional procedure to deliver the MNPs to the tumor site.[90] Moreover, MNPs remain in the brain around the delivery site for weeks to months, potentially allowing for multiple MHT sessions to be performed after a single delivery of MNPs.[89,91,92] Heating MNPs can also be precisely regulated by adjusting AMF parameters, and MHT produces a more uniform temperature distribution across brain lesions when compared with other thermal therapies such as LITT.[26,93] MHT provides a locally confined, remotely controllable, and easily reproducible form of HT.

PRECLINICAL APPLICATIONS OF MAGNETIC HYPERTHERMIA THERAPY IN NEUROSURGERY

Burton and colleagues[94] introduced the idea of applying a magnetic induction heating device to the brain using a ferromagnetic material. Since then, numerous preclinical studies have been conducted on brain cancer cell lines in vitro and in vivo primarily to (1) study efficacy, safety, and mechanism of action of MHT,[55,95–113] (2) develop and test new, more efficient and effective MHT nanoconstructs,[35,95–100,102,108–110,112,114–117] (3) assess MHT in combination with other therapies for brain cancer,[35,97,100,102,103,115,116,118] and (4) exploit the multifunctionality of MNPs for diagnostic and therapeutic applications.[35,47,97,100,103,115,116,119–122]

Although MHT is a highly localized form of HT, the nature of heat transfer makes spatial containment of energy deposition challenging, forcing further innovation. As a result, many researchers have focused on designing MNP constructs that heat well at non-toxic concentrations and target brain tumor cells for cancer-specific heating. One group showed that MIONPs encapsulated within positively charged liposomes had a high affinity for negatively charged glioma cells and generated intracellular hyperthermia in vitro that caused total cancer cell death after 40 min of MHT.[96] Another group used a calcium phosphate coating to increase MIONP internalization by GBM cell lines. They showed that allowing cancer cells to ingest the MIONPs for 24 h before AMF exposure significantly reduced cancer cell viability compared to when the AMF was applied immediately after MIONP administration but before internalization.[98] In addition, carboxymethyl-stevioside-modified magnetic dots demonstrating significant heating ability showed a profound anti-proliferative, anti-migratory, and anti-invasive effect on rodent glioma cells by inhibiting matrix metalloproteinase-2 and -9 expression, cell cycle arrest in the G0/G1 phase, and inducing oxidative stress upon re-exposure to an AMF.[95] These cancer cell-targeted applications of MNPs, and by extension MHT, may allow for lower concentrations of MNPs and lower power AMFs to be used for MHT. This is especially important when treating brain cancer due to the sensitivity of the brain and the potentially devastating effects that can occur from non-specific heating or MNP-related toxicity.

To further explore the clinical potential of MHT, several studies have focused on the possible synergism between MNPs/MHT and therapies currently used to treat HGGs. TMZ-loaded superparamagnetic NPs enhanced the cytotoxic effects of RT with a dose enhancement factor of 1.65.[103] In addition, this group showed that the combination of MHT, CT (TMZ), and RT caused enhanced anticancer efficacy compared to any monotherapy or two-modality combination therapy. Another group designed a temporary 2-5 cm balloon implant capable of being filled with MNPs and delivering high-dose rate brachytherapy for concurrent MHT and RT. They found that when using a human head phantom, they could heat tissue around the brain resection cavity at-risk for residual cancer cell presence between 40°C and 48°C and improve the uniformity of heating over previous multi-catheter interstitial approaches.[118] Many other groups have shown that MNPs can be effective drug carriers for CT and showed an added anti-tumor effect when giving MHT in combination with CT.[35,100,103,115,116] Finally, MHT in combination with photothermal therapy (PTT) was shown to be more effective than either monotherapy.[102] The therapies complement one another since although MHT is not limited by depth, it produces less heat per NP compared to PTT. On the contrary, PTT is limited by the depth penetration of the near-infrared light used to generate heat but can generate higher temperatures than MHT.[102]

Another interesting field of research is the use of bacteria-derived magnetosomes in lieu of chemically synthesized MNPs for MHT.[99,108–110] Magnetotactic bacteria naturally synthesize magnetic iron oxide nanocrystals (magnetosomes) which, once purified and processed to remove harmful endotoxins, have excellent size, morphology, biocompatibility, and magnetic properties. Magnetosomes were shown to be more cytotoxic to cancer cells than healthy cells and had a higher antitumor efficacy than chemically synthesized MIONPs resulting in complete glioma tumor regression in some cases. This improved efficacy was likely because magnetosomes required lower AMF amplitude for effective MHT, displayed higher SLP, exhibited a less scattered distribution intratumorally, and were able to maintain tumor temperatures at 43-46°C for longer duration when compared to MIONPs at an equal iron concentration. Although magnetosomes offer several advantages over synthetic MNPs for MHT, their time-consuming and costly synthesis currently limits large-scale application.[123]

In addition to studying the ways in which various nanoconstructs can be applied for MHT, researchers have also focused on how MNPs may be used as dual therapeutic and diagnostic, or "theranostic," agents for brain cancer. Notably, MIONPs produce the highest relaxivity of magnetic resonance imaging (MRI) contrast agents known today, and numerous studies show that MNPs are effective MRI contrast agents when conjugated with cancer-specific moieties.[47,103,119] Similarly, one group found that systemically delivering MIONPs loaded into tumor-associated macrophages led to preferential accumulation of MIONPs at the tumor margin in rat gliomas, allowing for effective therapy and a clear delineation of the tumor border by multimodal imaging techniques.[122]

Optimal implementation of MHT requires verification of localization and persistence of the nanoparticles over time. Although MRI can be used for in vivo imaging of MIONPs, an emerging tomographic tracer imaging technique called magnetic particle imaging (MPI) offers many advantages over current MRI technology.[29] Briefly, MPI systems image MIONPs by generating strong magnetic field gradients. Within these gradients is a region of low magnetic field strength, known as the field-free point (FFP). As the FFP crosses a region containing MIONPs, the ensuing change in magnetization generates a signal that is used to create a high-resolution three-dimensional (3D) image by rastering the FFP through the sample volume, with no background signal from the tissue.[124–126] In a recent study, MPI showed higher sensitivity to detect MIONP-labeled cells than MRI and detected and quantified as few as 1×10^4 MIONP-labeled cancer cells dispersed throughout a mouse brain ex vivo.[120] Another advantage of MPI over MRI is that MPI can image MIONPs at concentrations typically used for MHT (50–100 mg of Fe per g of tissue). By contrast, when MIONPs exceed concentrations of 10^{-3} g Fe/g of tissue, they create a susceptibility artifact appearance on MRI that appears as a "black hole" that obscures tissue anatomy.[29] Further study of MPI is currently underway and has the potential to significantly advance the future clinical application of MHT.

CLINICAL APPLICATIONS OF MAGNETIC HYPERTHERMIA THERAPY IN NEUROSURGERY

Several clinical studies, both in the United States and internationally, have evaluated the use of MHT in human glioma patients. Characteristics of some are outlined in **Table 1**. Among the earliest was the study conducted by Iacono and colleagues,[127–129] which included a phase I clinical trial using adjuvant MHT in addition to RT in patients with either primary or recurrent HGGs (GBM or anaplastic astrocytoma). Twenty-eight patients received intratumoral nickel-4 wt.% silicon alloy ferromagnetic wire implants before 1 (11 patients) or 2 (17 patients) 60-min MHT sessions. The study found a median overall survival of 20.6 months, including 14.9-month overall survival for patients with GBM. Important to note in this safety trial were the three major complications found, including hydrocephalus secondary to edema from catheter implantation, pneumocephalus from failure to suture all scalp wounds after removal of the catheters, and intracranial hemorrhage at the time of catheter implantation. In addition, one patient died from treatment-related edema, who in retrospect was found to have too high of a ferromagnetic implant volume leading to a protocol change. In the cohort of 28 patients, 11 minor complications were observed, ranging from focal seizures to cerebral edema to neurological deficits. All minor complications were managed conservatively. The investigators were able to show a treatment response, with over 60% of temperature sensors in the tumor core, 35% of sensors at the tumor margin, and 3.5% of sensors in surrounding normal tissue exceeding 42°C. However, no significant difference was observed between the survival of patients in which tumor core temperatures exceeded 41.5°C and those in which lower temperatures were recorded. The authors concluded that although MHT in combination with RT may be an effective treatment option, significant morbidities were associated with this combination therapy. To better assess the effect of MHT, Stea and colleagues[130] conducted a

Table 1
Summarizing results from six clinical studies investigating magnetic hyperthermia therapy in combination with radiation therapy in high-grade gliomas patients with either primary or recurrent cancer.

Author (Year)	Journal (PMID)	Title	Primary Conclusion
Kobayashi et al,[131] 1991	J. Neurooncol. PMID: 1654402	Interstitial hyperthermia of malignant brain tumors by implant heating system: clinical experience	Safe and repeated MHT was possible in 23 out of 25 patients with malignant brain tumors with an overall response rate of 34.8%. No major side effects were observed. Degeneration of tumor cells, hemorrhage, vascular stasis, and thrombosis were seen in treated tumors adjacent to areas of coagulative necrosis around the ferromagnetic implant.
Stea et al,[128] 1992	Int. J. Radiat. Oncol. Biol. Phys PMID: 1429088	Treatment of malignant gliomas with interstitial irradiation and hyperthermia	Interstitial MHT of brain tumors with ferromagnetic implants is feasible and carries significant but acceptable morbidity given the extremely poor prognosis of this patient population. Preliminary survival analysis showed patients had a median survival of 20.6 months from diagnosis.
Stea et al,[130] 1994	Int. J. Radiat. Oncol. Biol. Phys PMID: 7928490	Interstitial irradiation versus interstitial thermoradiotherapy for supratentorial malignant gliomas: a comparative survival analysis	Multivariate analysis showed that MHT conferred a positive survival benefit as an adjuvant to RT. No difference was found in survival between 13 recurrent cancer patients treated with RT alone and 8 patients treated with MHT and RT.
Maier-Hauff et al,[51] 2007	J. Neurooncol. PMID: 16773216	Intracranial Thermotherapy using Magnetic Nanoparticles Combined with External Beam Radiotherapy: Results of a Feasibility Study on Patients with Glioblastoma Multiforme	MHT was generally well tolerated by all patients with minor or no side effects and signs of local tumor control were observed.
Maier-Hauff et al,[87] 2011	J. Neurooncol. PMID: 20845061	Efficacy and safety of intratumoral thermotherapy using magnetic iron-oxide nanoparticles combined with external beam radiotherapy on patients with recurrent glioblastoma multiforme	No serious complications were observed from thermotherapy using MNPs in combination with a reduced radiation dose. In 59 patients with recurrent GBM, MHT in combination with RT led to longer median overall survival following recurrence (mOS = 13.4 months, 95% CI: 10.6–16.2 months) compared with conventional therapies.

(continued on next page)

Table 1 (continued)			
Author (Year)	**Journal (PMID)**	**Title**	**Primary Conclusion**
Grauer et al,[90] 2019	J. Neurooncol. PMID: 30506500	Combined intracavitary thermotherapy with iron oxide nanoparticles and radiotherapy as a local treatment modality in recurrent glioblastoma patients	Intracavitary MHT combined with RT can induce a prominent inflammatory reaction around the resection cavity that might trigger potent antitumor immune responses.

follow-up study comparing MHT with RT to RT alone in patients with both primary and recurrent HGGs. In this study, multivariate analysis revealed that MHT conferred a positive survival benefit as an adjuvant to RT in patients with primary HGGs. However, in a subset of patients exhibiting recurrent tumors before treatment, the combination therapy provided no additional survival benefit compared to RT monotherapy.

Several international clinical studies were conducted over three decades to determine the effect of MHT, and to identify potential shortcomings of the intervention. In the early 1990s, Kobayashi and colleagues[131] performed between 10 and 46 sessions of MHT over a period of up to 23 weeks in 23 patients with malignant brain tumors. They found an overall response rate of 34.8% and reported nearly a doubling of response rate between untreated versus recurrent tumors (58.3% vs 30%). Patients tolerated the procedure well in this study, but the authors reported heterogenous temperature distribution and implant migration as potential limitations. In a smaller study of fourteen recurrent and two primary GBM patients, Maier-Hauff and colleagues[51] found that patients safely tolerated 4-10 (median 6) MHT sessions in combination with fractionated RT, and observed local tumor control. Rather than implanting ferromagnetic alloys through catheters (as had previously been performed by others), they directly implanted a high concentration (112 mg of Fe/mL) of aminosilane-coated MIONPs suspended in water into the tumor area. The same group conducted a larger trial of 59 patients with recurrent GBM in a two-center study in 2011 and reported a median overall survival from diagnosis of first tumor recurrence and from primary tumor diagnosis in the entire study population of 13.5 months (95% CI: 10.6–16.2) and 23.2 months (95% CI: 17.2–29.2), respectively.[87] Toxicity was relatively mild, and the most common symptoms observed during MHT were fever, headache, mild hypertension and tachycardia, and focal convulsions. Fourteen patients experienced transient worsening of their

preexisting hemiparesis. Drawbacks of MHT reported from this study included the need to remove all metal from the treatment area (including metal dental implants), and indefinite exclusion of MRI for subsequent diagnosis of tumor progression. The results of this study led to European approval of MHT in 2012 as an adjuvant therapy for recurrent GBM in combination with RT.[87]

In a recent study, six patients diagnosed with recurrent GBM received intracavitary thermotherapy following 5-ALA-guided tumor resection. After resection, the cavity wall was coated with two to three layers of MIONPs using a hydroxycellulose mesh and fibrin glue that increased MNP stability and generated higher local MNP concentrations.[90] All patients received six semi-weekly sessions of MHT (60 min each) followed by RT in four out of six patients. Of the four patients who received combination therapy, two showed durable treatment responses of more than 23 months. Median progression-free survival was 6.25 months and median overall survival was 8.15 months. Histopathological analysis revealed sustained necrosis without tumor activity in areas adjacent to IONPs, as well as an immune response with macrophage infiltration and CD3+ T cells. Patients experienced minor symptoms such as sweating and headaches. Edema was found in the surrounding MNP area in all cases (independent of RT), and all patients required postoperative dexamethasone, with four patients requiring MIONPs to be removed due to the significant nanoparticle-associated edema. The authors concluded that intracavitary MHT with RT induces a strong inflammatory response, including an antitumoral immune response, which may provide stabilization for recurrent GBM patients.

DISCUSSION

MHT has shown great promise in both preclinical and clinical studies for the treatment of HGGs. Preclinically, MHT can induce profound antitumor effects and synergism with CT and RT when used to treat HGGs. Furthermore, MNPs have been used as multifunctional agents in applications such as cancer-targeting drug carriers, MRI contrast agents, and as mediators of MHT. With respect to clinical applications, six studies conducted between 1988 and 2019 highlight the various applications, advantages, and shortcomings of MHT over the course of its use in neurosurgery. Ni-Si ferromagnetic wires, aminosilane-coated MIONPs, and Fe-Pt alloy implant seeds have all been used to study MHT in combination with RT in a total of 157 malignant brain tumor patients diagnosed with primary or recurrent cancer. Although median temperatures achieved in the tumors ranged from 42°C to 53.2°C across five studies, temperatures in individual patients reached as high as 82°C, highlighting extreme variations in heating likely due to differences in MIONP properties, inhomogeneous distribution or migration of magnetic materials, and/or poorly regulated application of the AMF across the lesion. Overall, these studies reported that MHT was well tolerated, conferred a survival benefit, and potentially induced an MHT-mediated antitumor immune response.

Although MHT is reported as well-tolerated, it is important to consider therapy-related toxicities seen in previous clinical trials, as surgeons consider future clinical applications of MHT. In the study conducted by Grauer and colleagues,[90] all six patients suffered significant perifocal edema around the MIONP deposits 2 to 5 months following treatment, and four patients required follow-up surgery to remove the MIONPs after which their symptoms improved. Focal seizures were also reported as a common side effect in many of the studies, though they were generally resolved with conservative management.[87,127,128] Separately, others reported toxicity related to the implantation of the catheters which were used to administer the ferromagnetic material and for thermometry.[127–129] One patient in the early phase of one of these studies died due to treatment-related edema. Notably, this patient had the greatest number of catheters ($n = 33$) implanted and received the highest volume (119 cm^3) of Ni-4 wt.% Si alloy ferromagnetic wires. A separate finding reported by Stea and colleagues[127–129] was the sharp temperature decrease at the tumor margin compared with the significantly higher temperatures achieved in the tumor core. Moreover, the authors found that when the ferromagnetic wires were spaced apart by 1.3 cm or more, the number of temperature sensors measuring 42°C in the tumor decreased by approximately 30%. More comprehensive edema management, prophylactic antiepileptics, improved MNP delivery methods for a more homogeneous distribution of MNPs, and better AMF treatment planning to reduce off-target heating in the brain should be implemented in future clinical trials.

Although MHT has many advantages, for MHT to achieve its full clinical potential it is crucial to know the MNP distribution and to perform real-time 3D thermometry in the region of interest. At present, there is no effective way to simultaneously visualize MIONPs and noninvasively measure temperatures in the tumor during MHT. MRI is often used for noninvasive thermometry with other HT modalities (ie, PTT); however, the high static magnetic fields of MRI inhibit MNP rotation needed for heat generation in MHT.[132,133] Furthermore, the susceptibility caused by MNPs prevents their use for MR thermometry. Currently, conventional thermometry during MHT is typically achieved by invasively inserting radio frequency-resistant fiber-optic temperature probes into the tumor. These probes provide measures of local average temperature, and their misplacement or movement during treatment causes misleading readings.[92] Although heating during MHT can be estimated for a given field amplitude and frequency, SLP, and MNP concentration, large thermal gradients and unexpected variations in heating result from inhomogeneous MNP distribution within the tumor.[92] Infrared thermometry,[134] ultrasound thermometry[135,136] and luminescent nanothermometry[137] are examples of noninvasive techniques developed to measure temperatures during MHT. However, each technique has its own challenges ranging from limitations in-depth penetration to inaccuracies in thermometry caused by body movement. Additional research is needed to assess the clinical potential of these techniques.[138]

Combining MHT with MPI promises to overcome many of the obstacles facing the clinical application of MHT. In addition to enabling direct visualization of MIONPs, the underlying physics of MPI can be applied to provide real-time, noninvasive magnetic nanothermometry (MNT) during MHT.[29] Current research focuses on designing a device to simultaneously perform real-time MNT and MPI, and to inform and modulate AMF amplitude and frequency throughout the region of interest during MHT for regulated and reproducible delivery of a predetermined thermal dose. Recent studies have investigated systems capable of dual MPI-MHT,[139] as well as MPI systems fit for human use in the brain.[140,141] Future clinical success of MHT depends on developing an integrated MPI–MNT–MHT system. Such a system has the potential to minimize patient toxicity seen in previous clinical trials that is possibly related to magnetic material migration and inhomogeneous heating.

FUTURE DIRECTIONS

The future of MHT as it relates to treating brain cancer is bright, although significant research is required for MHT to become a widely implemented clinical therapy in the treatment of HGGs. The reported survival benefits, general tolerability, and potential anti-tumor immune effect in response to MHT in combination with RT seen in clinical trials all warrant future investigation. It is important that future clinical studies account for variables that may affect clinical outcomes, such as ethnicity and preexisting comorbidities, as previous studies did not account for those variables. In addition, most clinical trials have assessed MHT in combination with RT, but few have fully explored MHT in combination with CT. Given the current standard of care for GBM, which consists of concomitant RT and TMZ CT, such studies are warranted. In addition, prior studies included small cohorts of patients, and future studies need to include larger patient populations, in addition to randomized controlled trials to compare MHT to current standard practices. Current clinical efforts include designing a phase-I study of recurrent GBM patients and assessing safety, tolerability, and clinical antitumor activity of MHT in 3 cohorts treated with predetermined thermal doses of 45°C, 50°C, and 55°C, respectively.[90]

Designing and studying biocompatible nanoconstructs made optimally for MHT, MPI, and MNT, as well as for synergism with current therapies for HGGs is a large field of research that needs further exploration. In addition, carefully designed translational and clinical studies are required to develop technology that enables concurrent MPI–MNT–MHT. These studies have the potential to dramatically improve what is already a highly localized and efficacious form of HT for the treatment of aggressive, therapy-resistant forms of brain cancer.

SUMMARY

In summary, MHT is a localized, repeatable, and remotely controllable form of HT that offers many benefits over current heat-based therapies used to treat brain cancer. Its use within neurosurgery spans decades and it has been implemented to treat HGGs in both preclinical and clinical studies. Although significant limitations remain for clinical applications of MHT, there is reason to be optimistic that future developments will overcome these shortcomings as MHT is reported to be generally tolerable and associated with overall survival benefits in glioma patients.[142] Maximizing the clinical potential of MHT requires integrating noninvasive thermometry, MNP imaging, and thermotherapy into a single platform such that volume and extent of heating can be confirmed. Overall, MHT has the potential to enhance current therapies used to treat HGGs as an adjuvant therapy and provide patients suffering from some of the most aggressive and therapy-resistant forms of cancer with improved quality of life and better outcomes.

CLINICS CARE POINTS

- Prophylactic antiepileptics, comprehensive edema management, and close monitoring/regulation of body temperature should be considered when administering magnetic hyperthermia therapy (MHT) to reduce side effects of focal convulsions, treatment-related edema, and generalized thermal stress.

- A multi-trajectory approach for the delivery of magnetic nanoparticles (MNPs) is imperative to promote the homogenous distribution of MNPs and heating throughout the lesion and tumor margin where infiltrating cancer cells reside.

- Real-time thermometry and magnetic particle imaging should be implemented during MHT to ensure that the appropriate thermal dose is being delivered to the region of interest.

CONFLICT OF INTERESTS

Dr C.G. Hadjipanayis is a consultant for Stryker Corp., Synaptive Medical, and Hemerion.

REFERENCES

1. Alumutairi L, Yu B, Filka M, et al. Mild magnetic nanoparticle hyperthermia enhances the susceptibility of Staphylococcus aureus biofilm to antibiotics. Int J Hyperthermia 2020;37(1):66–75.

2. Gao X, Chen H. Hyperthermia on skin immune system and its application in the treatment of human papillomavirus-infected skin diseases. Front Med 2014;8(1):1–5. Epub 2014/01/10.

3. Roussakow S, editor. The history of hyperthermia rise and decline. Conference papers in science. London UK; USA: Hindawi; John Wiley & Sons; 2013.

4. Attaluri A, Kandala SK, Wabler M, et al. Magnetic nanoparticle hyperthermia enhances radiation therapy: a study in mouse models of human prostate cancer. Int J Hyperthermia 2015;31(4):359–74.

5. Gunderson LL, Tepper JE. Clinical radiation oncology. USA: Elsevier Health Sciences; 2015.

6. Kalamida D, Karagounis IV, Mitrakas A, et al. Fever-range hyperthermia vs. hypothermia effect on cancer cell viability, proliferation and HSP90 expression. PLoS One 2015;10(1):e0116021.

7. van der Zee J. Heating the patient: a promising approach? Ann Oncol 2002;13(8):1173–84.

8. Fajardo LF, Egbert B, Marmor J, et al. Effects of hyperthermia in a malignant tumor. Cancer 1980; 45(3):613–23.

9. Moon SD, Ohguri T, Imada H, et al. Definitive radiotherapy plus regional hyperthermia with or without chemotherapy for superior sulcus tumors: a 20-year, single center experience. Lung Cancer 2011;71(3):338–43.

10. Kampinga HH. Cell biological effects of hyperthermia alone or combined with radiation or drugs: a short introduction to newcomers in the field. Int J Hyperthermia 2006;22(3):191–6.

11. Pu P-y, Zhang Y-z, Jiang D-h. Apoptosis induced by hyperthermia in human glioblastoma cell line and murine glioblastoma. Chin J Cancer Res 2000;12(4):257–62.

12. Lee Titsworth W, Murad GJ, Hoh BL, et al. Fighting fire with fire: the revival of thermotherapy for gliomas. Anticancer Res 2014;34(2):565–74.

13. Man J, Shoemake JD, Ma T, et al. Hyperthermia Sensitizes Glioma Stem-like Cells to Radiation by Inhibiting AKT Signaling. Cancer Res 2015;75(8): 1760–9.

14. Ando K, Suzuki Y, Kaminuma T, et al. Tumor-specific CD8-positive T cell-mediated antitumor immunity is implicated in the antitumor effect of local hyperthermia. Int J Hyperthermia 2018;35(1):226–31.

15. den Brok MHMGM, Sutmuller RPM, van der Voort R, et al. In situ tumor ablation creates an antigen source for the generation of antitumor immunity. Cancer Res 2004;64(11):4024–9.

16. Salehi A, Paturu MR, Patel B, et al. Therapeutic enhancement of blood-brain and blood-tumor barriers permeability by laser interstitial thermal therapy. Neurooncol Adv 2020;2(1):vdaa071.

17. Tabatabaei SN, Girouard H, Carret A-S, et al. Remote control of the permeability of the blood–brain barrier by magnetic heating of nanoparticles: A proof of concept for brain drug delivery. J Control Release 2015;206:49–57.

18. Skitzki JJ, Repasky EA, Evans SS. Hyperthermia as an immunotherapy strategy for cancer. Curr Opin Investig Drugs 2009;10(6):550–8. Epub 2009/06/ 11. PubMed PMID: 19513944; PMCID: PMC2 828267.

19. Kozissnik B, Bohorquez AC, Dobson J, et al. Magnetic fluid hyperthermia: advances, challenges, and opportunity. Int J Hyperthermia 2013;29(8):706–14.

20. Dennis CL, Ivkov R. Physics of heat generation using magnetic nanoparticles for hyperthermia. Int J Hyperthermia 2013;29(8):715–29.

21. Gavilán H, Simeonidis K, Myrovali E, et al. How size, shape and assembly of magnetic nanoparticles give rise to different hyperthermia scenarios. Nanoscale 2021;13(37):15631–46.

22. Soetaert F, Kandala SK, Bakuzis A, et al. Experimental estimation and analysis of variance of the measured loss power of magnetic nanoparticles. Sci Rep 2017;7(1):6661. Epub 2017/07/29. PubMed PMID: 28751720; PMCID: PMC5532265 patents, including those describing BNF- and JHU-nanoparticle formulations. All patents are assigned to Johns Hopkins University, micromod Partikeltechnologie, GmbH, or Aduro Biotech, Inc. All other authors declare no competing interests.

23. Lanier OL, Korotych OI, Monsalve AG, et al. Evaluation of magnetic nanoparticles for magnetic fluid hyperthermia. Int J Hyperthermia 2019;36(1): 686–700.

24. Cleveland R, Sylvar D, Ulcek J. Evaluating compliance with FCC guidelines for human exposure to radio frequency electromagnetic fields. In: OET bulletin 65, UFC commission. US Federal Communications Commission Office of Engineering & Technology; 1997. p. 11–4.

25. Périgo EA, Hemery G, Sandre O, et al. Fundamentals and advances in magnetic hyperthermia. Appl Phys Rev 2015;2(4):041302.

26. Soetaert F, Korangath P, Serantes D, et al. Cancer therapy with iron oxide nanoparticles: Agents of thermal and immune therapies. Adv Drug Deliv Rev 2020;163-164:65–83.

27. Jain TK, Reddy MK, Morales MA, et al. Biodistribution, clearance, and biocompatibility of iron oxide magnetic nanoparticles in rats. Mol Pharm 2008;5(2):316–27.

28. Thakor AS, Jokerst JV, Ghanouni P, et al. Clinically approved nanoparticle imaging agents. J Nucl Med 2016;57(12):1833–7.

29. Healy S, Bakuzis AF, Goodwill PW, et al. Clinical magnetic hyperthermia requires integrated magnetic particle imaging. WIREs Nanomedicine and Nanobiotechnology 2022;14(3):e1779.

30. Alromi DA, Madani SY, Seifalian A. Emerging Application of Magnetic Nanoparticles for Diagnosis and Treatment of Cancer. Polymers (Basel) 2021; 13(23). https://doi.org/10.3390/polym13234146.

31. Bulte JW, Kraitchman DL. Iron oxide MR contrast agents for molecular and cellular imaging. NMR Biomed 2004;17(7):484–99.

32. Zhu L, Ma J, Jia N, et al. Chitosan-coated magnetic nanoparticles as carriers of 5-fluorouracil:

preparation, characterization and cytotoxicity studies. Colloids Surf B Biointerfaces 2009;68(1):1–6.

33. Hua MY, Liu HL, Yang HW, et al. The effectiveness of a magnetic nanoparticle-based delivery system for BCNU in the treatment of gliomas. Biomaterials 2011;32(2):516–27.

34. Carvalho SM, Leonel AG, Mansur AAP, et al. Bifunctional magnetopolymersomes of iron oxide nanoparticles and carboxymethylcellulose conjugated with doxorubicin for hyperthermo-chemotherapy of brain cancer cells. Biomater Sci 2019;7(5):2102–22.

35. Liu F, Wu H, Peng B, et al. Vessel-targeting nanoclovers enable noninvasive delivery of magnetic hyperthermia-chemotherapy combination for brain cancer treatment. Nano Lett 2021;21(19):8111–8.

36. Torres-Lugo M, Rinaldi C. Thermal potentiation of chemotherapy by magnetic nanoparticles. Nanomedicine (Lond). 2013;8(10):1689–707.

37. Khochaiche A, Westlake M, O'Keefe A, et al. First extensive study of silver-doped lanthanum manganite nanoparticles for inducing selective chemotherapy and radio-toxicity enhancement. Mater Sci Eng C 2021;123:111970.

38. Auerbach M, Ballard H. Clinical use of intravenous iron: administration, efficacy, and safety. Hematology 2010;2010(1):338–47.

39. Danielson BG. Structure, chemistry, and pharmacokinetics of intravenous iron agents. J Am Soc Nephrol 2004;15(Suppl 2):S93–8.

40. Markides H, Rotherham M, Haj AJE. Biocompatibility and toxicity of magnetic nanoparticles in regenerative medicine. J Nanomater 2012;2012:Article 13.

41. Laurent S, Burtea C, Thirifays C, et al. Crucial ignored parameters on nanotoxicology: the importance of toxicity assay modifications and "cell vision". PLoS One 2012;7(1):e29997.

42. Mahmoudi M, Laurent S, Shokrgozar MA, et al. Toxicity evaluations of superparamagnetic iron oxide nanoparticles: cell "vision" versus physicochemical properties of nanoparticles. ACS Nano 2011;5(9):7263–76.

43. Dewey WC. Arrhenius relationships from the molecule and cell to the clinic. Int J Hyperthermia 1994;10(4):457–83.

44. Perlstein B, Ram Z, Daniels D, et al. Convection-enhanced delivery of maghemite nanoparticles: Increased efficacy and MRI monitoring. Neuro Oncol 2008;10(2):153–61.

45. Hadjipanayis CG, Machaidze R, Kaluzova M, et al. EGFRvIII Antibody–Conjugated Iron Oxide Nanoparticles for Magnetic Resonance Imaging–Guided Convection-Enhanced Delivery and Targeted Therapy of Glioblastoma. Cancer Res 2010;70(15):6303–12.

46. Bobo RH, Laske DW, Akbasak A, et al. Convection-enhanced delivery of macromolecules in the brain. Proc Natl Acad Sci U S A 1994;91(6):2076–80.

47. Shevtsov MA, Yakovleva LY, Nikolaev BP, et al. Tumor targeting using magnetic nanoparticle Hsp70 conjugate in a model of C6 glioma. Neuro Oncol 2014;16(1):38–49.

48. Zhou P, Zhao H, Wang Q, et al. Photoacoustic-Enabled Self-Guidance in Magnetic-Hyperthermia Fe@Fe3O4 Nanoparticles for Theranostics In Vivo. Adv Healthc Mater 2018;7(9):1701201.

49. Jia G, Han Y, An Y, et al. NRP-1 targeted and cargo-loaded exosomes facilitate simultaneous imaging and therapy of glioma in vitro and in vivo. Biomaterials 2018;178:302–16.

50. Alexiou C, Jurgons R, Schmid RJ, et al. Magnetic Drug Targeting—Biodistribution of the Magnetic Carrier and the Chemotherapeutic agent Mitoxantrone after Locoregional Cancer Treatment. J Drug Target 2003;11(3):139–49.

51. Maier-Hauff K, Rothe R, Scholz R, et al. Intracranial Thermotherapy using Magnetic Nanoparticles Combined with External Beam Radiotherapy: Results of a Feasibility Study on Patients with Glioblastoma Multiforme. J Neuro-Oncology 2007;81(1):53–60.

52. Gilchrist RK, Medal R, Shorey WD, et al. Selective inductive heating of lymph nodes. Ann Surg 1957;146(4):596–606.

53. Hu R, Ma S, Li H, et al. Effect of magnetic fluid hyperthermia on lung cancer nodules in a murine model. Oncol Lett 2011;2(6):1161–4.

54. Kossatz S, Grandke J, Couleaud P, et al. Efficient treatment of breast cancer xenografts with multifunctionalized iron oxide nanoparticles combining magnetic hyperthermia and anti-cancer drug delivery. Breast Cancer Res 2015;17(1):66.

55. Jordan A, Scholz R, Maier-Hauff K, et al. The effect of thermotherapy using magnetic nanoparticles on rat malignant glioma. J Neurooncol 2006;78(1):7–14.

56. Zhao Q, Wang L, Cheng R, et al. Magnetic nanoparticle-based hyperthermia for head & neck cancer in mouse models. Theranostics 2012;2(1):113–21.

57. Wang L, Dong J, Ouyang W, et al. Anticancer effect and feasibility study of hyperthermia treatment of pancreatic cancer using magnetic nanoparticles. Oncol Rep 2012;27(3):719–26.

58. Johannsen M, Gneveckow U, Thiesen B, et al. Thermotherapy of prostate cancer using magnetic nanoparticles: feasibility, imaging, and three-dimensional temperature distribution. Eur Urol 2007;52(6):1653–61.

59. Johannsen M, Gneveckow U, Taymoorian K, et al. Morbidity and quality of life during thermotherapy using magnetic nanoparticles in locally recurrent

prostate cancer: results of a prospective phase I trial. Int J Hyperthermia 2007;23(3):315–23.

60. Johannsen M, Thiesen B, Wust P, et al. Magnetic nanoparticle hyperthermia for prostate cancer. Int J Hyperthermia 2010;26(8):790–5.

61. Johannsen M, Gneveckow U, Eckelt L, et al. Clinical hyperthermia of prostate cancer using magnetic nanoparticles: presentation of a new interstitial technique. Int J Hyperthermia 2005; 21(7):637–47.

62. AANS. Glioblastoma Multiforme, Available at: https://www.aans.org/Patients/Neurosurgical-Conditions-and-Treatments/Glioblastoma-Multiforme, 2019. Accessed September 1, 2022.

63. Patel AP, Tirosh I, Trombetta JJ, et al. Single-cell RNA-seq highlights intratumoral heterogeneity in primary glioblastoma. Science 2014;344(6190): 1396–401.

64. Ostrom QT, Gittleman H, Xu J, et al. CBTRUS Statistical Report: Primary Brain and Other Central Nervous System Tumors Diagnosed in the United States in 2009–2013. Neuro-Oncology 2016; 18(suppl_5):v1–75.

65. Stupp R, Mason WP, van den Bent MJ, et al. Radiotherapy plus Concomitant and Adjuvant Temozolomide for Glioblastoma. N Engl J Med 2005;352(10): 987–96.

66. Sanai N, Polley M-Y, McDermott MW, et al. An extent of resection threshold for newly diagnosed glioblastomas 2011;115(1):3.

67. Ostrom QT, Patil N, Cioffi G, et al. CBTRUS Statistical Report: Primary Brain and Other Central Nervous System Tumors Diagnosed in the United States in 2013-2017. Neuro Oncol 2020; 22(Supplement_1):iv1–96.

68. Vehlow A, Cordes N. DDR1 (discoidin domain receptor tyrosine kinase 1) drives glioblastoma therapy resistance by modulating autophagy. Autophagy 2019;15(8):1487–8.

69. Shergalis A, Bankhead A 3rd, Luesakul U, et al. Current challenges and opportunities in treating glioblastoma. Pharmacol Rev 2018;70(3):412–45.

70. Safari M, Khoshnevisan A. Cancer stem cells and chemoresistance in glioblastoma multiform: a review article. J Stem Cells 2015;10(4):271–85.

71. Gerard CS, Straus D, Byrne RW. Surgical Management of Low-Grade Gliomas. Semin Oncol 2014; 41(4):458–67.

72. Díez Valle R, Hadjipanayis CG, Stummer W. Established and emerging uses of 5-ALA in the brain: an overview. J Neurooncol 2019;141(3):487–94.

73. Lan X, Jörg DJ, Cavalli FMG, et al. Fate mapping of human glioblastoma reveals an invariant stem cell hierarchy. Nature 2017;549(7671):227–32.

74. Lathia JD, Mack SC, Mulkearns-Hubert EE, et al. Cancer stem cells in glioblastoma. Genes Dev 2015;29(12):1203–17.

75. Sneed PK, Stauffer PR, McDermott MW, et al. Survival benefit of hyperthermia in a prospective randomized trial of brachytherapy boost +/- hyperthermia for glioblastoma multiforme. Int J Radiat Oncol Biol Phys 1998;40(2):287–95.

76. Corry PM, Robinson S, Getz S. Hyperthermic effects on DNA repair mechanisms. Radiology 1977;123(2):475–82.

77. Ihara M, Takeshita S, Okaichi K, et al. Heat exposure enhances radiosensitivity by depressing DNA-PK kinase activity during double strand break repair. Int J Hyperthermia 2014;30(2):102–9.

78. Nytko KJ, Thumser-Henner P, Russo G, et al. Role of HSP70 in response to (thermo)radiotherapy: analysis of gene expression in canine osteosarcoma cells by RNA-seq. Sci Rep 2020;10(1): 12779.

79. Khurana N, Laskar S, Bhattacharyya MK, et al. Hsp90 induces increased genomic instability toward DNA-damaging agents by tuning down RAD53 transcription. Mol Biol Cell 2016;27(15): 2463–78.

80. Corry PM, Dewhirst MW. Thermal medicine, heat shock proteins and cancer. Int J Hyperthermia 2005;21(8):675–7.

81. van den Tempel N, Zelensky AN, Odijk H, et al. On the Mechanism of Hyperthermia-Induced BRCA2 Protein Degradation. Cancers (Basel) 2019;11(1). https://doi.org/10.3390/cancers11010097.

82. Krawczyk PM, Eppink B, Essers J, et al. Mild hyperthermia inhibits homologous recombination, induces BRCA2 degradation, and sensitizes cancer cells to poly (ADP-ribose) polymerase-1 inhibition. Proc Natl Acad Sci U S A 2011;108(24):9851–6.

83. Ko SH, Ueno T, Yoshimoto Y, et al. Optimizing a Novel Regional Chemotherapeutic Agent against Melanoma: Hyperthermia-Induced Enhancement of Temozolomide Cytotoxicity. Clin Cancer Res 2006;12(1):289–97.

84. Marino A, Camponovo A, Degl'Innocenti A, et al. Multifunctional temozolomide-loaded lipid superparamagnetic nanovectors: dual targeting and disintegration of glioblastoma spheroids by synergic chemotherapy and hyperthermia treatment. Nanoscale 2019;11(44):21227–48.

85. Yang X, Gao M, Xu R, et al. Hyperthermia combined with immune checkpoint inhibitor therapy in the treatment of primary and metastatic tumors. Front Immunol 2022;13. https://doi.org/10.3389/fimmu.2022.969447.

86. Yan B, Liu C, Wang S, et al. Magnetic hyperthermia induces effective and genuine immunogenic tumor cell death with respect to exogenous heating. J Mater Chem B 2022;10(28):5364–74.

87. Maier-Hauff K, Ulrich F, Nestler D, et al. Efficacy and safety of intratumoral thermotherapy using magnetic iron-oxide nanoparticles combined with

external beam radiotherapy on patients with recurrent glioblastoma multiforme. J Neurooncol 2011; 103(2):317–24.

88. Bouras A, Kaluzova M, Hadjipanayis CG. Radiosensitivity enhancement of radioresistant glioblastoma by epidermal growth factor receptor antibody-conjugated iron-oxide nanoparticles. J Neurooncol 2015;124(1):13–22.

89. Kaluzova M, Bouras A, Machaidze R, et al. Targeted therapy of glioblastoma stem-like cells and tumor non-stem cells using cetuximab-conjugated iron-oxide nanoparticles. Oncotarget 2015;6(11): 8788–806.

90. Grauer O, Jaber M, Hess K, et al. Combined intracavitary thermotherapy with iron oxide nanoparticles and radiotherapy as local treatment modality in recurrent glioblastoma patients. J Neurooncol 2019;141(1):83–94.

91. Platt S, Nduom E, Kent M, et al. Canine model of convection-enhanced delivery of cetuximab-conjugated iron-oxide nanoparticles monitored with magnetic resonance imaging. Clin Neurosurg 2012;59:107–13.

92. Jordan A. Hyperthermia classic commentary: 'Inductive heating of ferrimagnetic particles and magnetic fluids: Physical evaluation of their potential for hyperthermia' by Andreas Jordan et al., International Journal of Hyperthermia, 1993;9:51–68. Int J Hyperthermia 2009;25(7):512–6.

93. Liu L, Ni F, Zhang J, et al. Thermal analysis in the rat glioma model during directly multipoint injection hyperthermia incorporating magnetic nanoparticles. J Nanosci Nanotechnol 2011;11(12): 10333–8.

94. Burton C, Hill M, Walker AE. The RF Thermoseed-A Thermally Self-Regulating Implant for the Production of Brain Lesions. IEEE Trans Biomed Eng 1971;18(2):104–9. BME-.

95. Gupta R, Sharma D. (Carboxymethyl-stevioside)-coated magnetic dots for enhanced magnetic hyperthermia and improved glioblastoma treatment. Colloids Surf B Biointerfaces 2021;205:111870.

96. Shinkai M, Yanase M, Honda H, et al. Intracellular hyperthermia for cancer using magnetite cationic liposomes: in vitro study. Jpn J Cancer Res 1996; 87(11):1179–83.

97. Yin PT, Shah BP, Lee KB. Combined magnetic nanoparticle-based microRNA and hyperthermia therapy to enhance apoptosis in brain cancer cells. Small 2014;10(20):4106–12.

98. Adamiano A, Wu VM, Carella F, et al. Magnetic calcium phosphates nanocomposites for the intracellular hyperthermia of cancers of bone and brain. Nanomedicine (Lond). 2019;14(10): 1267–89.

99. Hamdous Y, Chebbi I, Mandawala C, et al. Biocompatible coated magnetosome minerals with various organization and cellular interaction properties induce cytotoxicity towards RG-2 and GL-261 glioma cells in the presence of an alternating magnetic field. J Nanobiotechnology 2017;15(1):74.

100. Zamora-Mora V, Fernández-Gutiérrez M, González-Gómez Á, et al. Chitosan nanoparticles for combined drug delivery and magnetic hyperthermia: From preparation to in vitro studies. Carbohydr Polym 2017;157:361–70.

101. Mamani JB, Marinho BS, Rego GNA, et al. Magnetic hyperthermia therapy in glioblastoma tumor on-a-Chip model. Einstein (Sao Paulo) 2020;18: eAO4954.

102. Anilkumar TS, Lu YJ, Chen JP. Optimization of the Preparation of Magnetic Liposomes for the Combined Use of Magnetic Hyperthermia and Photothermia in Dual Magneto-Photothermal Cancer Therapy. Int J Mol Sci 2020;21(15). https://doi.org/ 10.3390/ijms21155187.

103. Minaei SE, Khoei S, Khoee S, et al. Sensitization of glioblastoma cancer cells to radiotherapy and magnetic hyperthermia by targeted temozolomide-loaded magnetite tri-block copolymer nanoparticles as a nanotheranostic agent. Life Sci 2022;306:120729.

104. Ito A, Shinkai M, Honda H, et al. Heat shock protein 70 expression induces antitumor immunity during intracellular hyperthermia using magnetite nanoparticles. Cancer Immunol Immunother 2003; 52(2):80–8.

105. Xu H, Zong H, Ma C, et al. Evaluation of nanomagnetic fluid on malignant glioma cells. Oncol Lett 2017;13(2):677–80.

106. Rego GNA, Mamani JB, Souza TKF, et al. Therapeutic evaluation of magnetic hyperthermia using Fe3O4-aminosilane-coated iron oxide nanoparticles in glioblastoma animal model. Einstein (Sao Paulo). 2019;17(4):eAO4786.

107. Rego GNA, Nucci MP, Mamani JB, et al. Therapeutic efficiency of multiple applications of magnetic hyperthermia technique in glioblastoma using aminosilane coated iron oxide nanoparticles: in vitro and in vivo study. Int J Mol Sci 2020;21(3). https://doi.org/10.3390/ijms21030958.

108. Alphandéry E, Idbaih A, Adam C, et al. Chains of magnetosomes with controlled endotoxin release and partial tumor occupation induce full destruction of intracranial U87-Luc glioma in mice under the application of an alternating magnetic field. J Control Release 2017;262:259–72. https://doi.org/10.1016/j.jconrel.2017.07.020.

109. Alphandéry E, Idbaih A, Adam C, et al. Development of non-pyrogenic magnetosome minerals coated with poly-l-lysine leading to full disappearance of intracranial U87-Luc glioblastoma in 100% of treated mice using magnetic hyperthermia. Biomaterials 2017;141:210–22.

110. Le Fèvre R, Durand-Dubief M, Chebbi I, et al. Enhanced antitumor efficacy of biocompatible magnetosomes for the magnetic hyperthermia treatment of glioblastoma. Theranostics 2017; 7(18):4618–31.

111. Yi GQ, Gu B, Chen LK. The safety and efficacy of magnetic nano-iron hyperthermia therapy on rat brain glioma. Tumour Biol 2014;35(3):2445–9.

112. Liu L, Ni F, Zhang J, et al. Silver nanocrystals sensitize magnetic-nanoparticle-mediated thermo-induced killing of cancer cells. Acta Biochim Biophys Sinica 2011;43(4):316–23.

113. Ohno T, Wakabayashi T, Takemura A, et al. Effective solitary hyperthermia treatment of malignant glioma using stick type CMC-magnetite. In vivo study. J Neurooncol 2002;56(3):233–9.

114. Meenach SA, Hilt JZ, Anderson KW. Poly(ethylene glycol)-based magnetic hydrogel nanocomposites for hyperthermia cancer therapy. Acta Biomater 2010;6(3):1039–46.

115. Zhao L, Yang B, Wang Y, et al. Thermochemotherapy mediated by novel solar-planet structured magnetic nanocomposites for glioma treatment. J Nanosci Nanotechnol 2012;12(2):1024–31.

116. Arriaga MA, Enriquez DM, Salinas AD, Garcia R Jr, et al. Application of iron oxide nanoparticles to control the release of minocycline for the treatment of glioblastoma. Future Med Chem 2021;13(21): 1833–43.

117. Jiang H, Wang C, Guo Z, et al. Silver nanocrystals mediated combination therapy of radiation with magnetic hyperthermia on glioma cells. J Nanosci Nanotechnol 2012;12(11):8276–81.

118. Stauffer PR, Rodrigues DB, Goldstein R, et al. Feasibility of removable balloon implant for simultaneous magnetic nanoparticle heating and HDR brachytherapy of brain tumor resection cavities. Int J Hyperthermia 2020;37(1): 1189–201.

119. Shevtsov MA, Nikolaev BP, Yakovleva LY, et al. Superparamagnetic iron oxide nanoparticles conjugated with epidermal growth factor (SPION-EGF) for targeting brain tumors. Int J Nanomedicine 2014;9:273–87.

120. Melo KP, Makela AV, Knier NN, et al. Magnetic microspheres can be used for magnetic particle imaging of cancer cells arrested in the mouse brain. Magn Reson Med 2022;87(1):312–22.

121. Luo Y, Yang J, Yan Y, et al. RGD-functionalized ultrasmall iron oxide nanoparticles for targeted T1-weighted MR imaging of gliomas. Nanoscale 2015;7(34):14538–46.

122. Wang S, Shen H, Mao Q, et al. Macrophage-Mediated Porous Magnetic Nanoparticles for Multimodal Imaging and Postoperative Photothermal Therapy of Gliomas. ACS Appl Mater Inter 2021; 13(48):56825–37.

123. Taher Z, Legge C, Winder N, et al. Magnetosomes and Magnetosome Mimics: Preparation, Cancer Cell Uptake and Functionalization for Future Cancer Therapies. Pharmaceutics 2021;13(3). https://doi.org/10.3390/pharmaceutics13030367.

124. Bulte JWM. Superparamagnetic iron oxides as MPI tracers: A primer and review of early applications. Adv Drug Deliv Rev 2019;138:293–301.

125. Gleich B, Weizenecker J. Tomographic imaging using the nonlinear response of magnetic particles. Nature 2005;435(7046):1214–7.

126. Wu LC, Zhang Y, Steinberg G, et al. A Review of Magnetic Particle Imaging and Perspectives on Neuroimaging. AJNR Am J Neuroradiol 2019; 40(2):206–12.

127. Stea B, Cetas TC, Cassady JR, et al. Interstitial thermoradiotherapy of brain tumors: preliminary results of a phase I clinical trial. Int J Radiat Oncol Biol Phys 1990;19(6):1463–71.

128. Stea B, Kittelson J, Cassady JR, et al. Treatment of malignant gliomas with interstitial irradiation and hyperthermia. Int J Radiat Oncol Biol Phys 1992; 24(4):657–67.

129. Iacono RP, Stea B, Lulu BA, et al. Template-guided stereotactic implantation of malignant brain tumors for interstitial thermoradiotherapy. Stereotact Funct Neurosurg 1992;59(1–4): 199–204.

130. Stea B, Rossman K, Kittelson J, et al. Interstitial irradiation versus interstitial thermoradiotherapy for supratentorial malignant gliomas: a comparative survival analysis. Int J Radiat Oncol Biol Phys 1994;30(3):591–600.

131. Kobayashi T, Kida Y, Tanaka T, et al. Interstitial hyperthermia of malignant brain tumors by implant heating system: clinical experience. J Neurooncol 1991;10(2):153–63.

132. Jordan A, Wust P, Fählin H, et al. Inductive heating of ferrimagnetic particles and magnetic fluids: Physical evaluation of their potential for hyperthermia. Int J Hyperthermia 1993;9(1):51–68.

133. Mehdaoui B, Carrey J, Stadler M, et al. Influence of a transverse static magnetic field on the magnetic hyperthermia properties and high-frequency hysteresis loops of ferromagnetic FeCo nanoparticles. Appl Phys Lett 2012;100(5):052403.

134. Rodrigues HF, Mello FM, Branquinho LC, et al. Real-time infrared thermography detection of magnetic nanoparticle hyperthermia in a murine model under a non-uniform field configuration. Int J Hyperthermia 2013;29(8):752–67.

135. Lewis MA, Staruch RM, Chopra R. Thermometry and ablation monitoring with ultrasound. Int J Hyperthermia 2015;31(2):163–81.

136. Hadadian Y, Uliana JH, Carneiro AAO, et al. A Novel Theranostic Platform: Integration of Magnetomotive and Thermal Ultrasound Imaging With

Magnetic Hyperthermia. IEEE Trans Biomed Eng 2021;68(1):68–77.

137. Ortgies DH, Teran FJ, Rocha U, et al. Optomagnetic Nanoplatforms for In Situ Controlled Hyperthermia. Adv Funct Mater 2018;28(11):1704434.

138. Rodrigues HF, Capistrano G, Bakuzis AF. In vivo magnetic nanoparticle hyperthermia: a review on preclinical studies, low-field nano-heaters, noninvasive thermometry and computer simulations for treatment planning. Int J Hyperthermia 2020; 37(3):76–99.

139. Tay ZW, Chandrasekharan P, Chiu-Lam A, et al. Magnetic Particle Imaging-Guided Heating in Vivo Using Gradient Fields for Arbitrary Localization of

Magnetic Hyperthermia Therapy. ACS Nano 2018; 12(4):3699–713.

140. Graeser M, Thieben F, Szwargulski P, et al. Human-sized magnetic particle imaging for brain applications. Nat Commun 2019;10(1):1936.

141. Borgert J, Schmidt JD, Schmale I, et al. Perspectives on clinical magnetic particle imaging. Biomed Tech (Berl) 2013;58(6):551–6.

142. Shirvalilou S, Khoei S, Esfahani AJ, et al. Magnetic Hyperthermia as an adjuvant cancer therapy in combination with radiotherapy versus radiotherapy alone for recurrent/progressive glioblastoma: a systematic review. J Neurooncol 2021;152(3): 419–28.

Current Applications of Ablative Therapies for Trigeminal Neuralgia

Arpan R. Chakraborty, MD[a,b], Kerrin Sunshine, MD[a,b],
Jonathan P. Miller, MD[a,b], Jennifer A. Sweet, MD[a,b],*

KEYWORDS

- Trigeminal neuralgia • Ablative therapies • Rhizotomy • Neurectomy • Radiosurgery

KEY POINTS

- There are many ablative therapies for patients with trigeminal neuralgia who fail medical management.
- Peripherally, nerve blocks and neurectomies can be performed for pain relief.
- At the Gasserian ganglion, rhizotomy has been proven effective to provide lasting relief.
- Stereotactic radiosurgery (SRS) and partial sensory rhizotomy are other options for ablative procedures.

BACKGROUND

Trigeminal neuralgia (TN) is defined as sudden, recurrent, electrical shock-like pain in one or more divisions of the trigeminal nerve unilaterally. TN affects 4 to 13 people per 100,000 people annually, with women being affected more than men.[1] The average age of onset in patients without multiple sclerosis is 50 to 60 years of age. Most cases of TN involve a single branch of the trigeminal nerve (maxillary or mandibular), whereas about a third of cases involve both the maxillary and mandibular branch. The ophthalmic branch is rarely involved, seen in less than 5% of cases. Increase in age is the biggest risk factor for developing TN. In patients with TN, pain attacks are often initiated by a trigger point (light touch and toothbrush) in the pattern of the nerve distribution. Each pain attack is followed by a brief refractory period. Pain attacks can occur very frequently to the point of debilitation.

The trigeminal nerve consists of three branches: V1 (ophthalmic, purely sensory), V2 (maxillary, purely sensory), and V3 (mandibular, sensory/motor). These nerves travel to the trigeminal ganglion (also known as Gasserian ganglion) in Meckel's cave. The trigeminal nerve then travels to the spinal trigeminal nucleus where they synapse with second-order neurons that then travel to the ventral posteromedial nucleus in the thalamus, which then relays information to the sensory cortex. Various therapies are targeted at different areas of this pathway to provide relief to patients with TN **Fig. 1**.

The pathophysiology of TN is thought to occur at the peripheral level, related to changes in nerve myelination and/or dysregulation of voltage-gated sodium channels (which explains the efficacy of medications that affect those channels. These changes may result from compression of the nerve, usually by the superior cerebellar artery, although the anterior inferior cerebellar artery, the vertebral artery, and the petrosal vein complex have also been implicated in cases of TN. Compression of the nerve usually occurs usually within a few millimeters of the root entry zone. For certain cases of TN, the cause of the pain can be due to other masses near the TN causing

a Department of Neurological Surgery, University Hospitals, Cleveland Medical Center, 11100 Euclid Avenue, HAN 5042, Cleveland, OH 44106, USA; b Case Western Reserve University, School of Medicine, Cleveland, OH, USA
* Corresponding author.
E-mail address: Jennifer.sweet@uhhospitals.org

Neurosurg Clin N Am 34 (2023) 285–290
https://doi.org/10.1016/j.nec.2022.12.005
1042-3680/23/© 2023 Elsevier Inc. All rights reserved.

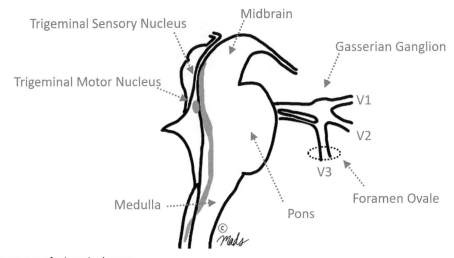

Fig. 1. Anatomy of trigeminal nerve.

nerve compression (meningioma, vascular malformations, epidermoid cysts, etc.)

TN is classified into classical, secondary, and idiopathic categories according to the International Classification of Headache Disorders, Third Edition (ICHD-3). Classical TN is related to vascular compression, whereas secondary TN results from structural causes of pain, including tumors or multiple sclerosis, and idiopathic cases are associated with no clear cause. TN can also be classified based on symptomology into Type 1 and Type 2 categories. Type 1 consists of paroxysmal pain either entirely (Type 1A) or with some component of constant pain (Type 1B), whereas type 2 consists of predominantly constant pain with some degree of paroxysmal pain (Type 2A) or in isolation (Type 2B).[2] According to ICHD-3, diagnosis of TN is clinically made with the following criteria[3].

A. Recurrent paroxysms of facial pain unilaterally that fulfills criteria B and C.
B. Pain has the following characteristics: can last a fraction of a second to approximately 2 minutes with severe intensity in an electric-shock-like or shooting characteristic
C. Innocuous stimuli can trigger pain in the stereotyped distribution
D. No alternative ICHD-3 diagnosis better explains the symptoms

When making the diagnosis of TN, it is often recommended to obtain a high-quality MRI of the brain to distinguish classical TN from secondary TN.

The first line of treatment of TN consists of medical management, including anti-epileptic medication such as carbamazepine or oxcarbazepine. These medications work via modulation of voltage-gated sodium channels that lead to a decrease in neuronal activity.[4] Carbamazepine, the first-line treatment, has approximately 70% effectiveness in symptom control.[4] Other medications that are used for the treatment of TN include baclofen, lamotrigine, phenytoin, gabapentin, clonazepam, and valproic acid.

For patients with radiographic evidence of vascular compression of the trigeminal nerve who do not respond to medical management, microvascular decompression is often considered for pain relief. This procedure is highly effective at providing relief, with long-term pain relief achieved in more than 80% of patients who undergo surgery.[5] However, in cases without evidence of neurovascular compression, or in patients who are poor surgical candidates, ablative therapies can be an effective treatment option.

DISCUSSION OF ABLATIVE THERAPIES

Ablative therapies are defined as procedures aimed at the destruction of the trigeminal nerve, which can be performed at different anatomic segments of the nerve. To be a candidate for ablative procedures, patients have failed medical management, often have symptoms of TN type 2 (ie, more constant pain than episodic), do not have evidence of neurovascular compression, or have findings that make them poor candidates for microvascular decompression (MVD), such as venous compression or prior MVD. Contraindication for ablative therapies, with the exception of tractotomies and DREZotomies, include patients with numbness in the distribution of the trigeminal nerve, favoring a diagnosis of trigeminal neuropathic pain or deafferentation pain.

Major treatments for TN at the peripheral anatomic level include cryotherapy, neurectomy, and alcohol injections. Cryotherapy consists of freezing the nerve at the infraorbital or mandibular foramen. The use of a cryoprobe causes a reversible ablation of the nerve leading to pain relief. Pain relief from this form of therapy has been observed to be 18 to 54 months. Cryotherapy is a relatively low-risk intervention that can be repeated as needed to provide pain relief. Neurectomy is another ablative procedure performed at the peripheral level. This is generally performed by accessing the infraorbital or inferior alveolar nerve via an intra-oral approach and avulsing the nerve. Often, material titanium screws or gold foil can be used to pack the foramen the nerves exit through to help with sustained avulsion of the nerve. This procedure is relatively well tolerated and can often be performed under local anesthesia. Relief of TN symptoms after peripheral neurectomy lasts 24 to 36 months.[6] Peripheral nerve block with alcohol injection, which can be performed under fluoroscopic guidance, is another ablative procedure that can be performed for refractory TN. Nerve blocks traditionally have been viewed as ineffective, although recent data suggests that permanent pain reduction is seen in about half of patients.[7]

At the level of the Gasserian ganglion, thermal radiofrequency rhizotomy, balloon compression rhizotomy, and glycerol rhizotomy are all effective treatment options for TN. All are performed by percutaneously advancing an instrument from the mandibular angle into the foramen ovale to target the Gasserian ganglion. The foramen ovale can be found with the use of anatomic landmarks and fluoroscopy, although neuronavigation can also be used. Haertel's landmarks are used to target the foramen, using an entry point 2 cm lateral and 1 cm inferior to the corner of the mouth and choosing a trajectory toward the intersection of the mid-pupillary line and tragus **Fig. 2**. Lateral fluoroscopy can be helpful the needle trajectory should be aimed at the junction between the line of the olfactory planum and the line of the clivus **Fig. 3**. A submental view can be used to directly visualize the foramen ovale, and lateral fluoroscopy provides information about needle depth. Return of spinal fluid and/or jaw jerk can help to confirm correct positioning. Once the location is verified, a lesion is produced.

Each option for rhizotomy has pros and cons. Thermal rhizotomy gives the surgeon the option of selective destruction to the mandibular and maxillary division of the trigeminal nerve it requires stimulation interaction with the patient to recreate patient's pain pattern and deliver the proper thermal dose. Glycerol rhizotomy is inexpensive and more useful for maxillary and mandibular pain. Balloon compression is more useful for multidivisional pain including first-division pain because the induced damage to the nerve is more widespread. Percutaneous rhizotomy is generally indicated for patients who have episodic, sharp facial pain. It is generally not recommended for patients with continuous facial pain. For all rhizotomy techniques, the most debilitating side effect is anesthesia dolorosa or deafferentation pain, which is defined as constant, severe facial pain in the setting of numbness in the distribution of the affected nerve **Fig. 4**.

Radiofrequency rhizotomy consists of the application of heat to the nerve, typically 60 to 90° Celsius for 60 to 90 s. Because thermal lesioning is very potent in comparison with other techniques, it is helpful to use test stimulation under awake anesthesia to verify the location in the desired branch of the nerve where the pain is located and adjusting the location within the trigeminal nerve to target the desired area. Probes with different curvatures can allow additional selectivity (a straight probe is best for targeting V2, whereas an upward curve can target V1 and a downward curve can target V3). In an analysis of over 1500 patients who underwent thermocoagulation of the Gasserian ganglion, 57.7% of patients were painless for 5 years and did not require oral medication.[8] At a 15-year follow-up, 42.2% of patients still had no recurrence of pain.[8] Complications from thermal rhizotomy include diminished corneal reflex, masseter weakness and paralysis, dysesthesia, keratitis, and cerebrospinal fluid leak. Minimization of risks is achieved by precise localization of foramen ovale. Thermal rhizotomy can be used not only for classical TN but also secondary and idiopathic, as opposed to microvascular decompression.

Glycerol rhizotomy uses chemical rather than thermal ablation. Once the foramen is accessed and spinal fluid return is obtained, up to 0.3 mL of glycerol is then injected to produce the lesion, after which the patient is then maintained in a semi-sitting position for 1 to 2 hours. Unlike thermal rhizotomy and balloon compression, where one can control the exact heat or pressure and duration, there is not an exact technique to target the precise distribution of the ablation, although smaller volumes will preferentially target lower divisions of the trigeminal nerve.

Balloon compression uses mechanical energy to create the ablation and requires general anesthesia due to the pain of the procedure. Like thermal rhizotomy, it is possible to target specific divisions of the trigeminal nerve by manipulating the position of the balloon, which is inflated at the desired location.

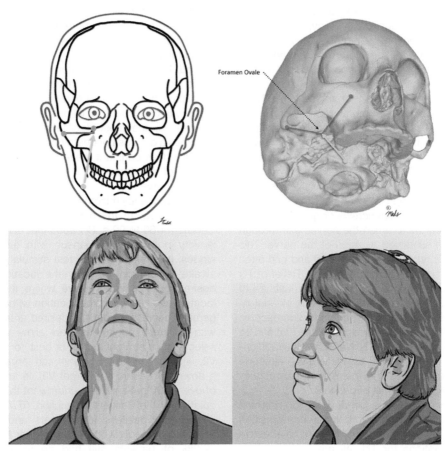

Fig. 2. Hartel's landmark. The needle (represented by the green line) enters the foramen ovale to target the gasserian ganlion. Its trajectory can be guided by facial landmarks, aligning with the midpupillary point and the anterior tragus (shown with blue lines).

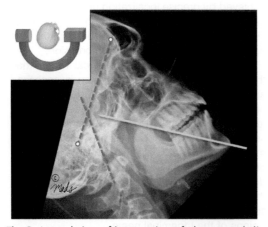

Fig. 3. Lateral view of intersection of planum and clivus. The needle (represented by the green line) enters the foramen ovale to target the gasserian ganlion. Its trajectory can also be guided by lateral radiographic landmarks, aiming for the point of intersection between the the line of the olfactory planum and the line of the clivus (shown with blue lines).

Balloon compression is thought to ablate large and small myelinated nerves responsible for TN with the preservation of unmyelinated fibers, which may preserve corneal sensation, and for this reason it is sometimes preferred for the treatment of ophthalmic division pain.[9] Balloon compression ranges across all three divisions treating pain across the entire nerve. This provides advantage over thermocoagulation where the probe must be repositioned to provide a wide range of relief. Balloon compression and glycerol injection can be performed under general anesthesia, which may be helpful if patients cannot tolerate awake procedures.

Various ablative treatment options also exist to treat TN at the root entry zone of the trigeminal nerve in the posterior fossa. Partial sensory rhizotomy technique such as internal neurolysis is a surgical option for patients who have refractory TN. It is performed using a retrosigmoid craniotomy to expose the nerve (a similar approach to MVD), which is then partially transected near the

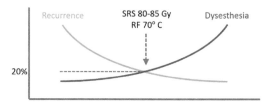

Fig. 4. Radiofrequency rhizotomy.

root entry zone to provide relief of pain along with loss of sensation. This treatment option may be helpful for patients who do not have significant vascular compression of the trigeminal nerve or vascular anatomy that makes MVD unsafe to perform. It can also be performed at the time of an MVD procedure to further increase the chances of long-lasting effects. Effectiveness of partial sensory rhizotomy is found to be about 40% to 60%, with about a third of patients having recurring symptoms.[10,11] Risks of the procedure are similar to those of MVD, with some literature citing a higher incidence of facial numbness after surgery.

Radiosurgery to the nerve root is another option that can provide relief of pain for some patients, including those with tolerable face pain refractory to medical management who cannot undergo surgical treatment or patients who have posterior fossa lesions as the source of their pain. Radiosurgery typically takes many weeks before pain relief is seen, so it is not recommended for patients who have severe pain and need immediate relief. Radiosurgery is performed with the use of a stereotactic head frame. High-resolution MRI is used to localize the trigeminal nerve and for surgical planning. Typically, a single 4-mm isocenter of radiation is placed at the trigeminal nerve root entry zone for a single total dose of 80 to 90 Gy (40–45 Gy at the 50% isodose line). The radiation can be targeted proximally at the dorsal root entry zone or distally at the retrogasserian zone, although more proximal lesions are associated with less sensory loss. For patients who have masses causing their pain, usually, the target will be the lesion instead of the nerve. In a retrospective analysis of over 500 patients treated with radiosurgery for TN, pain relief was achieved in 73% at 1 year, 65% at 2 years, and 41% at 5 years.[1] Radiation delivery takes approximately 30 to 60 minutes, and SRS is typically done as an outpatient.

Brainstem lesioning procedures such as trigeminal tractotomy or nucleotomy are not typically performed for TN but can be helpful for other kinds of facial neuropathic pain. These procedures are performed at the level of the spinal

trigeminal nucleus and trigeminal tract. They can be done via an open surgical approach, or percutaneously via image guidance. When performed percutaneously, a needle is positioned with stereotactic guidance. Sensory and motor stimulation is tested and then ablation is performed. In a similar fashion, ablative procedures can be performed at the dorsal root entry zone (also known as DREZotomy). DREZotomy is usually performed for deafferentation pain. The nucleus caudalis is the target of this approach. For nucleus caudalis DREZotomy, a C1 hemilaminectomy or laminectomy is performed for access. The C2 rootlet, obex, sulcus intermediolateralis and cranial roots of the accessory nerve are landmarks used by the surgeon during surgery to localize the area to be targeted. Lesioning is performed by an electrode above the sensory rootlets of the C2 within the intermediolateral sulcus above the obex. The probe is held perpendicular to the medualla and around 20 lesions can be created between the obex and C2 nerve root. This is performed with intraoperative monitoring. In one longitudinal analysis of nucleus caudalis DREZotomy, 60% of patients reported pain relief 1 year after the procedure. Reports of transient ataxia and hemiparesis are reported as morbidity of the procedure.[12]

SUMMARY

TN can be a debilitating pain syndrome that is often refractory to medical management. Although surgical therapy often consists of microvascular decompression when there is radiographic evidence of neurovascular compression of the trigeminal nerve, several ablative therapies are also an option for appropriately selected patients. Ablative therapies consist of techniques that injure the nerve to provide pain relief. To date, there are no large trials comparing the myriad of ablative therapies to elucidate if any has a clear benefit over the other. Instead, specific therapies must be tailored to the individual. In general, less invasive therapies such as peripheral nerve blocks, rhizotomies of the Gasserian ganglion, or radiosurgery of the root entry zone can offer effective pain relief via minimally invasive techniques for patients who do not exhibit sensory deficits consistent with trigeminal neuropathic pain or deafferentation pain. These procedures can often be repeated as needed if patients experience periodic relief of their symptoms without numbness or anesthesia dolorosa. More invasive procedures such as partial sensory rhizotomy and DREZotomy require surgical exposure to perform and thus carry more morbidity and mortality.

CLINICS CARE POINTS

- The etiology of trigeminal neuralgia (TN) has not been definitively established, but many cases are associated with compression of the trigeminal nerve by a blood vessel at the trigeminal root entry zone adjacent to the brainstem
- Ablative treatment options are appropriate for both TN of unknown etiology as well as ones associated with TN compression
- Inclusion criteria for ablative therapies: typically patients with symptoms of TN type 2 who have failed medical management, have no neurovascular compression on imaging, have findings that make MVD less favorable, such as venous compression or prior MVD, or patients who are poor surgical candidates for open surgical procedures
- Exclusion criteria for ablative therapies (with the exception of tractotomies and DREZotomies): patients with numbness in the distribution of the trigeminal nerve consistent with trigeminal neuropathic pain or deafferentation pain
- Possible side effects from ablative therapies include weakness of muscles of mastication, cranial nerve deficits, meningitis, dysesthesias, anesthesia dolorosa, corneal numbness, and keratitis
- Ablative therapies should be targeted to provide the longest duration of pain relief while reducing the risk of these side effects, as these are not only debilitating but can be prohibitive of subsequent treatments

DISCLOSURE

None of the authors has any conflict of interest to disclose.

REFERENCES

1. Kondziolka D, Zorro O, Lobato-Polo J, Kano H, Flannery TJ, Flickinger JC, et al. Gamma Knife stereotactic radiosurgery for idiopathic trigeminal neuralgia. J Neurosurg 2010;112:758–65.

2. Burchiel K. A new classification for facial pain. Neurosurgery 2003;53:1164–7.

3. The international classification of headache disorders: 2nd edition. Cephalalgia 2004;24(Suppl 1):9–160.

4. Gambeta E, Chichorro JG, Zamponi GW. Trigeminal neuralgia: An overview from pathophysiology to pharmacological treatments. Mol Pain 2020;16. 1744806920901890.

5. Maarbjerg S, Di Stefano G, Bendtsen L, Cruccu G. Trigeminal neuralgia – diagnosis and treatment. Cephalalgia 2017;37:648–57.

6. Ali FM, Prasant M, Pai D, Aher VA, Kar S, Safiya T. Peripheral neurectomies: A treatment option for trigeminal neuralgia in rural practice. J Neurosci Rural Pract 2012;3:152–7.

7. Han KR, Chae YJ, Lee JD, Kim C. Trigeminal nerve block with alcohol for medically intractable classic trigeminal neuralgia: long-term clinical effectiveness on pain. Int J Med Sci 2017;14:29–36.

8. Kanpolat Y, Savas A, Bekar A, Berk C. Percutaneous Controlled Radiofrequency Trigeminal Rhizotomy for the Treatment of Idiopathic Trigeminal Neuralgia: 25-year Experience with 1600 Patients. Neurosurgery 2001;48:524–34.

9. Brown JA. 30 Percutaneous Ablative Treatment of Neuropathic Facial Pain. In: Gross RE, Boulis NM, editors. Neurosurgical operative atlas: functional neurosurgery. 3rd Edition. New York, New York: Thieme Medical Publishers, Inc.; 2018.

10. Xia L, Zhong J, Zhu J, Wang YN, Dou NN, Liu MX, et al. Effectiveness and safety of microvascular decompression surgery for treatment of trigeminal neuralgia: a systematic review. J Craniofac Surg 2014;25:1413–7.

11. Young JN, Wilkins RH. Partial sensory trigeminal rhizotomy at the pons for trigeminal neuralgia. J Neurosurg 1993;79:680–7.

12. Kanpolat Y, Tuna H, Bozkurt M, Elhan AH. Spinal and nucleus caudalis dorsal root entry zone operations for chronic pain. Oper Neurosurg 2008;62:235–44.

Pros and Cons of Ablation for Functional Neurosurgery in the Neurostimulation Age

Marwan Hariz, MD, PhD*

KEYWORDS

- Ablative surgery • Deep brain stimulation • Parkinson disease • Tremor radiofrequency
- Pallidotomy • Thalamotomy • Focused ultrasound

KEY POINTS

- Radiofrequency ablation (thalamotomy, pallidotomy) was the main treatment of Parkinson disease (PD) until the advent of Levodopa in the 1970s, after which it declined.
- Starting in the mid-1980s, unilateral radiofrequency posteroventral pallidotomy heralded the renaissance of surgery for PD and became the first efficient ablative procedure for advanced PD to carry level-one evidence.
- Deep brain stimulation (DBS) has been the dominating functional neurosurgery procedure in the last 2 decades, allowing safe bilateral simultaneous surgery but DBS incurred high costs and stricter patient selection than ablation, and resulted in lack of training of younger generations of neurosurgeons in performing radiofrequency ablations.
- Ablative neurosurgery is experiencing a renaissance in part thanks to introduction of focused ultrasound and in part due to the drawbacks of long-term DBS.
- Especially for movement disorders, ablative neurosurgery using radiofrequency coagulation is still needed but lacks sponsorship and industry promotion.

BACKGROUND/INTRODUCTION

Both ablative procedures of subcortical structures and neurostimulation emerged in parallel at the dawn of stereotactic functional neurosurgery.[1] For both procedures, the first applications were in the realm of psychiatry[1–3] and then in pain and epilepsy and thereafter overwhelmingly in movement disorders.[1,4] Both surgical methods have known ups and downs during their 70+ years history but for different reasons.

In psychiatry, both neurostimulation and ablation declined soon after their introduction, due to the general backlash against lobotomy and all psychiatric surgery in the late 1960s and 1970s, coupled with the introduction of several brands of antipsychotic medications, and, in parallel, the increase of psychodynamic psychiatry—as opposed to biological psychiatry. This decline of all psychiatric neurosurgery has still not recovered despite the many efforts of functional neurosurgeons to promote Deep brain stimulation (DBS) as a lenient alternative to stereotactic ablation in surgical treatment of obsessive compulsive disorder (OCD) and depression.[5,6]

In the realm of movement disorders, initial attempts to promote DBS were doomed due to the cumbersomeness of the technique and the nonavailability of fully implantable neuro-pacemakers.[4] It is first in the late 1980s, when implantable pulse generators became available, that the modern neurostimulation age started, initially targeting the ventral intermediate nucleus (VIM) of the thalamus for the treatment of tremor.[7]

Department of Clinical Neuroscience, University Hospital, Umeå 90185, Sweden
* Corresponding author. UCL-Queen Square Institute of Neurology, London WC1N 3BG.
E-mail addresses: marwan.hariz@umu.se; m.hariz@ucl.ac.uk

Neurosurg Clin N Am 34 (2023) 291–299
https://doi.org/10.1016/j.nec.2022.11.006
1042-3680/23/© 2022 Elsevier Inc. All rights reserved.

Ablative surgery for movement disorders, especially PD, had its first long-lasting honeymoon in the 1950s and 1960s, using mainly radiofrequency (RF) coagulation as the safe and versatile method par excellence to produce stereotactic lesions. With the advent of Levodopa in the late 1960s, thalamotomies and pallidotomies for PD became almost extinguished. Ablative surgery witnessed a new world-wide renaissance with the reintroduction of Leksell's posteroventral pallidotomy in the early 1990s[8–10] for the treatment of the postlevodopa PD but declined then sharply at the turn of the new millennium due to the emergence of DBS of the subthalamic nucleus (STN) and the globus pallidus internus (GPi).[11] Meanwhile, DBS in the VIM of the thalamus in the treatment of essential and other tremors had almost completely overshadowed the previous thalamotomy.[12]

Recently, a new dawn of ablative surgery is slowly reemerging due partly to the introduction of Laser Interstitial Thermo Therapy (LITT),[13,14] and especially the promotion of "incision-less" ablative techniques enabled by MR-guided focused ultrasound (MRgFUS) to produce focused deep brain ablations,[15] and also by the Leksell Gammaknife (LGK) to make radiosurgical thalamotomies for tremor.[16] Hence, the neurosurgical armamentarium available today for functional stereotactic procedures comprises the neurostimulation technique based on DBS (and dorsal column stimulation, DCS, which will not be dealt with in this article) and ablative surgery using either RF, LITT, LGK or MRgFUS. Even though functional neurosurgery is still at present well entrenched into the "neurostimulation" age and much dominated by DBS,[17,18] there may be a resurgence for ablative surgery, partly driven by the introduction of tools allowing surgery without skull opening (especially MrgFUS) and where "fashion"[19] as well as other interests[20] may play a role.

Although there are very few head-to-head comparisons between stereotactic neuroablation and neurostimulation, from the point of view of the patient referred to surgery, a sober evaluation and weighing of the pros and cons of each technique for a particular condition is what ultimately matters.

Functional neurosurgery for pain has been addressed in previous issues of Neurosurgical Clinics,[21,22] and epilepsy surgery was comprehensively addressed in Neurosurgical Clinics Volume 31, Issue 3: Epilepsy Surgery: The Network Approach Edited by Vasileios Kokkinos, R. Mark Richardson, Pages H1-H6, 301 to 480 (July 2020). Therefore, this article will concentrate on pros and cons of ablation versus stimulation in the domains of psychiatric illness and movement disorders.

ABLATION VERSUS NEUROSTIMULATION FOR OBSESSIVE COMPULSIVE DISORDER AND DEPRESSION

Historically, anterior cingulotomy and anterior capsulotomy have been the most common ablative procedures, although rarely used. Ablation of these targets relied on RF coagulation and, in some cases of capsulotomy, on the Leksell gamma-knife.[23–25] Only recently, capsulotomy was performed with MRgFUS [26,27] and most recently with LITT.[14,28] Judging from the number of publications, the use of capsulotomy and cingulotomy have decreased greatly since the 1960s, reflecting the general downfall of psychiatric surgery, owing to the legacy of the previous lobotomy era. However, despite modern conservative management, there remain a substantial number of patients with OCD or depression who need surgery. The introduction of DBS in psychiatry was thought to mitigate societal and other negative attitudes toward surgery but despite a frenetic activity of DBS for OCD since 1999,[29] and of DBS for depression since 2005,[30] and with DBS eventually tried on a multitude of brain targets,[31] DBS has still not made a dent in psychiatry, as illustrated by a the appeal published recently in Nature Medicine.[6] At same time, ablative surgery in psychiatry is still considered taboo by many despite the fact that it has proven its efficacy and safety compared with DBS. Several recent reviews of both old and recent literature on ablation versus DBS in OCD have come to practically the same conclusions: that bilateral anterior capsulotomy is indeed efficient for OCD[32–34] and for depression,[35] and does not harbor more complications than DBS. It is therefore difficult to see the added-on clinical rational for use of DBS in surgical treatment of refractory OCD and depression, other than an attempt to circumvent the generally negative attitude toward stereotactic ablative psychosurgery, by presenting DBS as separate from surgery, such as illustrated in a publication from Harvard where one could read: "Treating obsessive-compulsive disorder. Options include medication, psychotherapy, surgery, and deep brain stimulation,"[36] as if DBS was something that does not involve surgery!

ABLATION VERSUS STIMULATION FOR PARKINSON'S DISEASE
Posteroventral Pallidotomy and Deep Brain Stimulation

In surgery for PD today, "ablation" means mainly pallidotomy and stimulation means DBS especially in the STN and the GPi. Starting in the mid-1990s,

Lauri Laitinen in Umea, Sweden, pioneered the renaissance of surgical treatment of PD by resurrecting "Leksell's posteroventral pallidotomy."[8–10,37] The basal ganglia model of PD subsequently provided the rational for the effects of posteroventral pallidotomy on the cardinal symptoms of PD,[38,39] and this procedure experienced a tremendous worldwide spread[40] and became the first evidence-based ablative surgical procedure for PD,[41] endorsed twice by the International Movement Disorders Society.[42,43] Although posteroventral pallidotomy was the most published surgical procedure for PD in the 1990s and early 2000, DBS in the pallidum and especially DBS in the STN DBS have all but supplanted it as preferred surgical methods for advanced PD because DBS can be done bilaterally, whereas pallidotomy or any other ablative surgery targeting the motor thalamus and basal ganglia can be safely performed only unilaterally. Thus, the main advantage of DBS compared with pallidotomy is that DBS allows bilateral and simultaneous surgery. Furthermore, DBS is adaptable permitting—within limits—to increase the current delivered when symptoms worsen and allows thanks to the quadripolar lead, to avoid or limit side effects. Finally, much has been said about the reversibility of DBS, even that DBS can be stopped or removed if needed but this is no longer valid after a long-time chronic DBS because of the risk for severe rebound of symptoms leading sometimes to death due to malignant parkinsonian or dystonic crisis.[44,45] In fact a new and dreadful diagnosis has emerged lately, labeled "DBS withdrawal syndrome."[46–48] This new and sometimes fatal syndrome can occur in some patients with Parkinson disease after long-term STN DBS or in some dystonia patients after long-term GPi DBS[49] when the battery is suddenly depleted and no replacement is available or affordable, or when hardware is explanted due to infection. In cases where such patients have been fortunate enough to receive a pallidotomy thanks to the neurosurgeons having been trained to perform this procedure, the sudden post-DBS deterioration was reversed by the pallidotomy.[50] Hence, RF pallidotomy seems to be a very potent procedure, provided it is done properly by experienced neurosurgeons (more on this in later discussion). In fact, previous blinded randomized studies of pallidotomy against best medical management have shown that at 2 years follow-up, pallidotomy yielded about 25% improvement of the off-medication scores of the Unified Parkinsońs Disease Rating scale (UPDRS9).[51,52]

Neurosurgeon Bob Gross from Emory University put it beautifully when he wrote: "unilateral pallidotomy is a relatively safe operation, compared with the benefits that can be expected. On its own merits, it is unlikely that modern pallidotomy would have been abandoned based on an excessive rate of adverse effects."[53] Hence, the demise of pallidotomy in the last 2 decades was neither due to its ineffectiveness on the symptoms of advanced PD, nor to excessive complications but for totally different reasons, some of which will be listed below.

Subthalamic Nucleotomy and Subthalamic Nucleus Deep Brain Stimulation

There is no doubt that today bilateral STN DBS is the main surgical procedure for PD, due mainly to its effectiveness in ameliorating the symptoms of PD, and to the fact that it is the only surgical procedure for PD that allows a radical decrease in medication dosage. The well-publicized neurological, behavioral, and other side effects of STN DBS, rather than contributing to slow down its popularity, have on the contrary contributed to expansion of DBS beyond PD, into the realm of psychiatry and behavior.[54,55]

No matter that STN DBS, when compared with any other surgical procedure for PD, requires the most stringent patient selection criteria, it still has great appeal to many clinicians and patients alike. For a long time, the STN was considered "no man's land" for lesional procedures because of the fear of inducing severe hyperkinesia and hemiballism but this dogma has been challenged.[56] A contemporary, extensive Cuban experience, involving evaluations by neurologists from Europe and the United States has shown that, in fact, stereotactic lesions of the STN, at least unilaterally, have resulted in a sustained good effect on PD symptoms, with low and acceptable risks of inducing violent dyskinesias.[57,58] Nonetheless, subthalamic nucleotomy remained rarely performed[59] but this may be about to change because of the introduction of MRgFUS. Indeed, a recent sham-controlled study by a Spanish team has shown that MRgFUS unilateral lesioning of the STN was feasible and efficient.[60] Why using MRgFUS lesioning of the STN would become more acceptable than using the good old RF lesioning remains a mystery.

ABLATION VERSUS STIMULATION FOR TREMOR

Ventrolateral thalamotomy, including VIM thalamotomy was for decades the most widespread surgical treatment of virtually all kinds of tremor (Parkinsonian, essential, dystonic, posttraumatic, MS, and so forth). However, thalamotomy could be performed safely only unilaterally. In 1987, when Benabid introduced VIM DBS contralateral to a previous thalamotomy,[7] he wrote: "VIM stimulation strongly decreased the tremor but failed to suppress it as completely as thalamotomy did." He attributed this to the stimulation frequency that was limited to 130 Hz. When eventually new generation of implantable neuropacemakers could deliver a frequency up to 185 HZ, the results improved, and VIM DBS became a firsthand procedure replacing thalamotomy, and it was shown that bilateral VIM DBS was feasible, efficient, and safe, which thalamotomy was not when done bilaterally. Hence RF thalamotomy was all but abandoned by functional neurosurgeons, especially after publication of a randomized study showing that both VIM DBS and VIM thalamotomy were efficient for control of tremor but that thalamotomy had more side effects and resulted in less improvement in quality of life than thalamic DBS.[61,62] However, further experience revealed that long time VIM DBS, particularly for essential tremor, could lead to problems with habituation, tolerance, and rebound of symptoms.[63,64]

Starting some 10 years ago, thalamotomy is experiencing a solid renaissance following the introduction of MRgFUS,[65] appealing to clinicians and patients alike because it allows surgery without opening of the skull. Hence, because of this new surgical tool, allowing incision-less surgery, VIM thalamotomy is expanding at the expenses of VIM DBS. Gone are the previous apprehensions that it is not good to "add a new lesion to an already sick brain."[66] Furthermore, there are ongoing trials aiming to show that MRgFUS allows even a staged *bilateral* VIM thalamotomy,[67] something that was taboo in the past.

ABLATION VERSUS STIMULATION FOR DYSTONIA

Historically, both thalamotomy and pallidotomy have been used to treat refractory dystonia.[10,68] Based on the excellent effect of Laitinen's posteroventral pallidotomy on Parkinsonian dyskinesias and dystonias, and following on the success of DBS as a method, surgery for dystonia in the last 2 decades has consisted overwhelmingly of DBS in the very same target used for pallidotomy, that is, in the posteroventral GPi. Notwithstanding this, there are indications that pallidotomy is being used as a rescue when patients experience symptom rebound following failure of DBS as well as in very severe cases of dystonic storm, including in pediatric patients.[69–71] In a patient with cervical dystonia, Blomstedt and colleagues[72] performed pallidotomy through the existing DBS electrode before its removal because of infection. The same procedure was reported in patients with generalized dystonia.[73] A recent article reported on a case of severe status dystonicus (SD) because of depleted DBS battery that could not be replaced.[49] The patient died despite intensive care treatment. Perhaps, a pallidotomy could have rescued that patient? Lately, there has been a resurgence of pallidotomy for various types dystonia, especially in Japan.[74–78] Recently, an article titled "Bilateral Pallidotomy for Dystonia: A Systematic Review" was published in Movement Disorders Journal by a Dutch team.[79] The authors conducted a systematic review of individual patient data concerning a total of 100 patients from 33 articles, including 25 patients with SD, in 23 of whom SD resolved after the bilateral pallidotomy. They concluded that "Given the burden of dystonia, bilateral pallidotomy should be regarded a viable tool in the armamentarium of the neurosurgeon in the treatment of dystonia, particularly for patients with contraindications for DBS or if the severity of the dystonic symptoms outweighs the risk of permanent speech disorders."

DISCUSSION

Undeniably, the last 20+ years—and ongoing—can be considered the "Neurostimulation Age," in which DBS is the absolutely dominating surgical procedure in functional stereotactic neurosurgery, both for movement disorders and for neuropsychiatric illness, and DBS is trialed in an increasing number of clinical indications and is explored on a multitude of "new" brain targets.[17,18] In parallel, stereotactic ablative surgery has been in sharp decline.

Reasons for the Popularity of Deep Brain Stimulation

The worldwide continuous popularity of deep brain stimulation has several reasons

DBS is indeed an efficient and somewhat low-risk therapy. DBS can be performed safely bilaterally on basal ganglia and thalamic targets; DBS is marketed as a "high-tech" and "reversible" procedure, even if this reversibility is perhaps not always valid in the long term; neurologists are increasingly in charge of, and enthusiastic about, DBS; DBS can be applied to, and trialed in any "novel" brain target, even targets not previously ablated (pedunculopontine nucleus, fornix), and even for conditions that have not been previously treated by ablative surgery (balance disturbances, Alzheimer dementia); there is a constant sponsorship from DBS manufacturers to scientific meetings and to various research program; industry is providing new and more sophisticated DBS hardware; there is ongoing sensational marketing in the media, as well as audiovisual promotion of DBS, especially on the Internet; a patient with implanted DBS electrodes is a convenient living human model for safe and ethical research in neuroscience; DBS allows to perform randomized controlled trials, in which stimulation can be double-blindly turned on or off (sham stimulation). Finally, a most important reason for the ongoing dominance of DBS is that neurosurgeons who know how to perform proper lesions are a disappearing species, and younger neurosurgeons have not been trained in the performance of stereotactic ablative surgery.[20]

Reasons for Decline of Stereotactic Ablations

In parallel to the above, reasons for decline of stereotactic ablative surgery include the following: young neurosurgeons are no longer trained in these procedures; lesions in thalamic and basal ganglia targets cannot be safely performed bilaterally simultaneously; it is not uncommon for some of the initial effects of stereotactic lesions to "wear off," which may involve the need for reoperation; "new" brain targets and some new indications may not be suitable for lesioning; neurologists are not as much "in control" in ablative surgery as in DBS; lesional procedures in psychiatric illness are not easily accepted owing to the legacy of the lobotomy era; in RF-based ablative surgery, there is no sponsorship from industry for research and for organization of scientific meetings; MRgFUS excepted, there is no sensational marketing or impressive audiovisual promotion on the Internet or in the lay press. Finally, there has been unfounded denigrations of lesional surgery, especially pallidotomy, still lingering until the present time,[80] and that some of those still in favor of ablative surgery are trying hard to counteract.[81] Nowhere are the reasons behind decline of RF lesions better illustrated than in this article from Oxford titled: "Expected Fate of Radiofrequency Lesioning: A Silent Death or a Cold-Blooded Murder."[20]

Why Ablative Surgery May Reemerge

Judging from the scholarly literature, we may be witnessing a renaissance of stereotactic lesioning, both in surgery for movement disorders and in psychiatry, thanks mainly to the introduction of MRgFUS and the application of GammaKnife radiosurgery in this field. MRgFUS has been Food and Drug Administration (FDA) approved for VIM thalamotomy in Essential and Parkinsonian tremor, as well as for pallidotomy in PD. It is trialed

for anterior capsulotomy in OCD and for some other applications. At the recently concluded congress of the World Society for Stereotactic and Functional Neurosurgery in Korea, there were more than 30 abstracts on MRgFUS.[82] Closed skull surgery, even called "incision-less" surgery is having a great appeal for patients and clinicians but this comes at a price: the machine is expensive; the whole hair of the patient has to be shaved; the procedure must be performed within the bore of the MRI machine, occupying it for several hours; there may be some limitations on conducting a proper neurological evaluation of the patient during lesioning; and not all skulls can accommodate MRgFUS depending on skull density ratio and depending on laterality of the brain target.[83] Notwithstanding these limitations, it looks like the reemergence of ablative surgery will be driven by the MRgFUS, which may spark a new interest in ablative surgery, including a renewed interest in the good old gold-standard RF thermocoagulation, and hence a renewed incentive among the young and future generations of functional neurosurgeons to learn its skills.

Pros and Cons of Ablation

What are the pros and cons of stereotactic ablation in the neurostimulation age?

An overview of the general advantages and disadvantages of stereotactic ablative surgery versus DBS is provided, regardless of the method of ablation being radiofrequency (RF) thermocoagulation, laser interstitial thermal therapy (LITT), MR-guided focused ultrasound, or radiosurgery using the LGK, regardless of indication, and regardless of brain targets (thalamotomy for tremor, posteroventral pallidotomy and subthalamic nucleotomy for advanced PD, thalamotomy or pallidotomy for dystonia, capsulotomy or cingulotomy for OCD and depression) (**Table 1**).

Pros: Compared with DBS, ablative surgery is much less expensive; shorter operation time; no foreign body; less risk for infection; no hardware issues; no cosmetic concerns; no "umbilical cord" between patient and DBS programmer requiring repetitive time-consuming postoperative adjustments of stimulation; can be done bilaterally and simultaneously in limbic targets such as anterior capsule and anterior cingulum for OCD and depression.

Cons: Compared with DBS in thalamus, pallidum, and STN in surgery for movement disorders, ablative surgery can only be performed unilaterally, and only occasionally bilaterally provided a staging of the 2 procedures; if lesion is misplaced, its side effects may be irreversible, or

Table 1
Pros and cons of ablative lesions versus deep brain stimulation

	Ablation	DBS
Efficacious	Yes	Yes
Selection criteria	Liberal	Stringent
Costs	Nonexpensive	Expensive
Need for targeting accuracy	Yes, very much	Yes
Wear-off of effect	Possible	Possible
Adaptability	No (unless redo surgery)	Yes, within limits
"Addictive"	No	Yes: "once DBS, always DBS"
Technique/training	Difficult	Less difficult
Severe complications	May happen	May happen
Side effects	*Usually* permanent	*Usually* adaptable
Reversibility of side effects	Usually not	Usually yes
Bilateral simultaneous	Possible in limbic targets, not in BG and T	Possible in all targets
Applicable on all targets	No	Yes
Applicable to all indications	No	Yes
"Acceptance" in psychiatry	Rarely	Sometimes
Postoperative workload	Minimal	Laborious
Risk for infection	No/negligible	Yes
Risk for hardware problems	—	Yes
Industry sponsorship and promotion	No (except for MRgFUS)	Yes
Allows sham	No (except MRgFUS and RS)	Yes
Denigrated sometimes	Yes	No
S U M M A R Y:	Still needed. Risk of lost skills…	Still expanding. Limited availability

Abbreviations: BG, basal ganglia; RS, radiosurgery; T, tremor.

only partly reversible; wear off of effect can occur needing a new operation; it receives no sponsorship by industry or audiovisual marketing (MRgFUS excepted); there is very limited possibility to perform sham surgery (MRgFUS excepted); and ablative surgery requires more training of neurosurgeons but, alas, training of younger generations of neurosurgeons in performing stereotactic ablation is lacking in most centers.

SUMMARY

Should one recommend stereotactic ablation for PD, tremor, dystonia and OCD, in this era of DBS? The answer depends on several variables such as the symptoms to treat, the patient's preferences and expectations, the surgeons' competence and preference, the availability of financial means (by government health care, by private insurance, and so forth), the geographical issues, and not least the current and dominating fashion at that particular time. Nevertheless, as shown in

Table 1, each technique has its pros and cons, and both ablation and stimulation can be either used alone or even combined (provided expertise in both of them) to treat various symptoms of movement and mind disorders in adequately selected patients.

CLINICS CARE POINTS

- RF ablative procedures in functional neurosurgery have fallen into oblivion in the last 2 decades following the spread and promotion of DBS.

- RF pallidotomy is an efficient, safe, and evidence-based surgery for advanced PD. Its demise was not due to an excessive rate of adverse effects.

- Ablative surgery is experiencing a renaissance in part thanks to introduction of focused ultrasound and in part due to the drawbacks of long-term DBS. There is a need for younger generations of functional neurosurgeons to learn or relearn the skills of ablative procedures.
- Especially for movement disorders, ablative surgery using RF coagulation, even if only unilateral, is still needed but lacks sponsorship and industry promotion.

DISCLOSURE

Nothing to disclose.

FUNDING

None.

REFERENCES

1. Hariz MI, Blomstedt P, Zrinzo L. Deep brain stimulation between 1947 and 1987: the untold story. Neurosurg Focus 2010;29(2):E1.
2. Rzesnitzek L, Hariz M, Krauss JK. Psychosurgery in the history of stereotactic functional neurosurgery. Stereotact Funct Neurosurg 2020;98(4):241–7.
3. Rzesnitzek L, Hariz M, Krauss JK. The origins of human functional stereotaxis: a reappraisal. Stereotact Funct Neurosurg 2019;97(1):49–54.
4. Blomstedt P, Hariz MI. Deep brain stimulation for movement disorders before DBS for movement disorders. Parkinsonism Relat Disord 2010;16(7): 429–33.
5. Widge AS, Deckersbach T, Eskandar EN, et al. Deep brain stimulation for treatment-resistant psychiatric illnesses: what has gone wrong and what should we do next? Biol Psychiatry 2016;79(4):e9–10.
6. Visser-Vandewalle V, Andrade P, Mosley PE, et al. Deep brain stimulation for obsessive-compulsive disorder: a crisis of access. Nat Med 2022;28(8): 1529–32.
7. Benabid AL, Pollak P, Louveau A, et al. Combined (thalamotomy and stimulation) stereotactic surgery of the VIM thalamic nucleus for bilateral Parkinson disease. Appl Neurophysiol 1987;50(1–6):344–6.
8. Laitinen LV, Bergenheim AT, Hariz MI. Leksell's posteroventral pallidotomy in the treatment of Parkinson's disease. J Neurosurg 1992;76(1):53–61.
9. Gildenberg PL. Evolution of basal ganglia surgery for movement disorders. Stereotact Funct Neurosurg 2006;84(4):131–5.
10. Cif L, Hariz M. Seventy years with the globus pallidus: pallidal surgery for movement disorders between 1947 and 2017. Mov Disord 2017;32(7):972–82.
11. The Deep-Brain Stimulation for Parkinson's Disease Study Group. Deep brain stimulation of the subthalamic nucleus or the pars interna of the globus pallidus in Parkinson's disease. N Engl J Med 2001; 345(13):956–63.
12. Tasker RR. Deep brain stimulation is preferable to thalamotomy for tremor suppression. Surg Neurol 1998;49(2):145–53.
13. Gross RE, Stern MA. Magnetic resonance guided stereotactic laser pallidotomy for dystonia. Mov Disord 2018;33(9):1502–3.
14. Satzer D, Mahavadi A, Lacy M, et al. Interstitial laser anterior capsulotomy for obsessive-compulsive disorder: lesion size and tractography correlate with outcome. J Neurol Neurosurg Psychiatr 2022;93(3): 317–23.
15. Bond AE, Shah BB, Huss DS, et al. Safety and efficacy of focused ultrasound thalamotomy for patients with medication-refractory, tremor-dominant Parkinson disease: a randomized clinical trial. JAMA Neurol 2017;74(12):1412–8.
16. Witjas T, Carron R, Krack P, et al. A prospective single-blind study of Gamma Knife thalamotomy for tremor. Neurology 2015;85(18):1562–8.
17. Harmsen IE, Wolff Fernandes F, Krauss JK, et al. Where are we with deep brain stimulation? A review of scientific publications and ongoing research. Stereotact Funct Neurosurg 2022;100(3):184–97.
18. Krauss JK, Lipsman N, Aziz T, et al. Technology of deep brain stimulation: current status and future directions. Nat Rev Neurol 2021;17(2):75–87.
19. Hariz M. Pallidotomy: a "Phoenix the Bird" of surgery for Parkinson's disease? Mov Disord Clin Pract 2022; 9(2):170–2.
20. Tripathi M, Aziz TZ. Expected fate of radiofrequency lesioning: a silent death or a cold-blooded murder. Stereotact Funct Neurosurg 2018;96(4):274–5.
21. Alamri A, Pereira EAC. Deep brain stimulation for chronic pain. Neurosurg Clin N Am 2022;33(3): 311–21.
22. Bao J, Tangney T, Pilitsis JG. Focused ultrasound for chronic pain. Neurosurg Clin N Am 2022;33(3): 331–8.
23. Lévêque M, Carron R, Régis J. Radiosurgery for the treatment of psychiatric disorders: a review. World Neurosurg 2013;80(3–4):S32.e1–9.
24. Spatola G, Martinez-Alvarez R, Martínez-Moreno N, et al. Results of Gamma Knife anterior capsulotomy for refractory obsessive-compulsive disorder: results in a series of 10 consecutive patients. J Neurosurg 2018;131(2):376–83.
25. Rasmussen SA, Noren G, Greenberg BD, et al. Gamma ventral capsulotomy in intractable obsessive-compulsive disorder. Biol Psychiatry 2018;84(5):355–64.
26. Davidson B, Hamani C, Rabin JS, et al. Magnetic resonance-guided focused ultrasound capsulotomy

for refractory obsessive compulsive disorder and major depressive disorder: clinical and imaging results from two phase I trials. Mol Psychiatry 2020; 25(9):1946–57.

27. Chang JG, Jung HH, Kim SJ, et al. Bilateral thermal capsulotomy with magnetic resonance-guided focused ultrasound for patients with treatment-resistant depression: a proof-of-concept study. Bipolar Disord 2020;22(7):771–4.

28. McLaughlin NCR, Lauro PM, Patrick MT, et al. Magnetic resonance imaging-guided laser thermal ventral capsulotomy for intractable obsessive-compulsive disorder. Neurosurgery 2021;88(6): 1128–35.

29. Nuttin B, Cosyns P, Demeulemeester H, et al. Electrical stimulation in anterior limbs of internal capsules in patients with obsessive-compulsive disorder. Lancet 1999;354(9189):1526.

30. Mayberg HS, Lozano AM, Voon V, et al. Deep brain stimulation for treatment resistant depression. Neuron 2005;45(5):651–60.

31. Krack P, Hariz MI, Baunez C, et al. Deep brain stimulation: from neurology to psychiatry? Trends Neurosci 2010;33(10):474–84.

32. Hageman SB, van Rooijen G, Bergfeld IO, et al. Deep brain stimulation versus ablative surgery for treatment-refractory obsessive-compulsive disorder: a meta-analysis. Acta Psychiatr Scand 2021;143(4): 307–18.

33. Pepper J, Hariz M, Zrinzo L. Deep brain stimulation versus anterior capsulotomy for obsessive-compulsive disorder: a review of the literature. J Neurosurg 2015;122(5):1028–37.

34. Pepper J, Zrinzo L, Hariz M. Anterior capsulotomy for obsessive-compulsive disorder: a review of old and new literature. J Neurosurg 2019;133(5): 1595–604.

35. Hurwitz TA, Honey CR, Sepehry AA. Ablation surgeries for treatment-resistant depression: a meta-analysis and systematic review of reported case series. Stereotact Funct Neurosurg 2022;1–14. https:// doi.org/10.1159/000526000.

36. Anonymous: treating obsessive-compulsive disorder. Options include medication, psychotherapy, surgery, and deep brain stimulation. Harv Ment Health Lett 2009;25:4–5.

37. Svennilson E, Torvik A, Lowe R, et al. Treatment of parkinsonism by stereotactic thermolesions in the pallidal region. A clinical evaluation of 81 cases. Acta Psychiatr Neurol Scand 1960;35(3):358–77.

38. Lang AE, Lozano AM. Parkinson's disease. First of two parts. N Engl J Med 1998;339(15):1044–53.

39. Lang AE, Lozano AM. Parkinson's disease. Second of two parts. N Engl J Med 1998;339(16): 1130–43.

40. Hariz MI. From functional neurosurgery to "interventional" neurology: a review of publications on thalamotomy, pallidotomy and DBS, between 1966 and 2001. Mov Disord 2003;18(8):845–52.

41. Goetz CG, Poewe W, Rascol O, et al. Evidence-based medical review update: pharmacological and surgical treatments of Parkinson's disease: 2001 to 2004. Mov Disord 2005;20(5):523–39.

42. Fox SH, Katzenschlager R, Lim SY, et al. The movement disorder society evidence-based medicine review update: treatments for the motor symptoms of Parkinson's disease. Mov Disord 2011;26(Suppl 3): S2–41.

43. Fox SH, Katzenschlager R, Lim SY, et al. International Parkinson and movement disorder society evidence-based medicine review: Update on treatments for the motor symptoms of Parkinson's disease. Mov Disord 2018;33(8):1248–66.

44. Hariz M. Once STN DBS, always STN DBS?–Clinical, ethical, and financial reflections on deep brain stimulation for Parkinson's disease. Mov Disord Clin Pract 2016;3(3):285–7.

45. Hariz M, Blomstedt P. Leksell's Posteroventral Pallidotomy 1992-2022: Quo Vadis? Stereotact Funct Neurosurg 2022;100(4):259–63.

46. Neuneier J, Barbe MT, Dohmen C, et al. Malignant deep brain stimulation-withdrawal syndrome in a patient with Parkinson's disease. Mov Disord 2013; 28(12):1640–1.

47. Reuter S, Deuschl G, Falk D, et al. Uncoupling of dopaminergic and subthalamic stimulation: life-threatening DBS withdrawal syndrome. Mov Disord 2015;30(10):1407–13.

48. Rajan R, Krishnan S, Kesavapisharady KK, et al. Malignant subthalamic nucleus deep brain stimulation withdrawal syndrome in Parkinson's disease. Mov Disord Clin Pract 2016;3(3):288–91.

49. Rohani M, Munhoz RP, Shahidi G, et al. Fatal status dystonicus in tardive dystonia due to depletion of deep brain stimulation's pulse generator. Brain Stimul 2017;10(1):160–1.

50. Bulluss KJ, Pereira EA, Joint C, et al. Pallidotomy after chronic deep brain stimulation. Neurosurg Focus 2013;35(5):E5.

51. Vitek JL, Bakay RA, Freeman A, et al. Randomized trial of pallidotomy versus medical therapy for Parkinson's disease. Ann Neurol 2003;53(5):558–69.

52. de Bie RM, de Haan RJ, Nijssen PC, et al. Unilateral pallidotomy in Parkinson's disease: a randomised, single-blind, multicentre trial. Lancet 1999; 354(9191):1665–9.

53. Gross RE. What happened to posteroventral pallidotomy for Parkinson's disease and dystonia? Neurotherapeutics 2008;5(2):281–93.

54. Mallet L, Polosan M, Jaafari N, et al. Subthalamic nucleus stimulation in severe obsessive-compulsive disorder. N Engl J Med 2008;359(20):2121–34.

55. Coenen VA, Honey CR, Hurwitz T, et al. Medial forebrain bundle stimulation as a pathophysiological

mechanism for hypomania in subthalamic nucleus deep brain stimulation for Parkinson's disease. Neurosurgery 2009;64(6):1106–14.

56. Guridi J, Obeso JA, Rodriguez-Oroz MC, et al. L-dopa-induced dyskinesia and stereotactic surgery for Parkinson's disease. Neurosurgery 2008;62(2):311–23.

57. Alvarez L, Macias R, Pavón N, et al. Therapeutic efficacy of unilateral subthalamotomy in Parkinson's disease: results in 89 patients followed for up to 36 months. J Neurol Neurosurg Psychiatry 2009;80(9): 979–85.

58. Ricardo Y, Pavon N, Alvarez L, et al. Long-term effect of unilateral subthalamotomy for Parkinson's disease. J Neurol Neurosurg Psychiatry 2019;90(12):1380–1.

59. Merello M, Tenca E, Pérez Lloret S, et al. Prospective randomized 1-year follow-up comparison of bilateral subthalamotomy versus bilateral subthalamic stimulation and the combination of both in Parkinson's disease patients: a pilot study. Br J Neurosurg 2008; 22(3):415–22.

60. Martínez-Fernández R, Máñez-Miró JU, Rodríguez-Rojas R, et al. Randomized trial of focused ultrasound subthalamotomy for Parkinson's disease. N Engl J Med 2020;383(26):2501–13.

61. Schuurman PR, Bosch DA, Bossuyt PM, et al. A comparison of continuous thalamic stimulation and thalamotomy for suppression of severe tremor. N Engl J Med 2000;342(7):461–8.

62. Schuurman PR, Bosch DA, Merkus MP, et al. Long-term follow-up of thalamic stimulation versus thalamotomy for tremor suppression. Mov Disord 2008; 23(8):1146–53.

63. Fasano A, Helmich RC. Tremor habituation to deep brain stimulation: Underlying mechanisms and solutions. Mov Disord 2019;34(12):1761–73.

64. Hariz MI, Shamsgovara P, Johansson F, et al. Tolerance and tremor rebound following long-term chronic thalamic stimulation for Parkinsonian and essential tremor. Stereotact Funct Neurosurg 1999; 72(2–4):208–18.

65. Elias WJ, Huss D, Voss T, et al. A pilot study of focused ultrasound thalamotomy for essential tremor. N Engl J Med 2013;369(7):640–8.

66. Krack P, Martinez-Fernandez R, Del Alamo M, et al. Current applications and limitations of surgical treatments for movement disorders. Mov Disord 2017; 32(1):36–52.

67. Iorio-Morin C, Yamamoto K, Sarica C, et al. Bilateral focused ultrasound thalamotomy for essential tremor (BEST-FUS phase 2 trial). Mov Disord 2021;36(11): 2653–62.

68. Cooper IS. 20-year followup study of the neurosurgical treatment of dystonia musculorum deformans. Adv Neurol 1976;14:423–52.

69. Marras CE, Rizzi M, Cantonetti L, et al. Pallidotomy for medically refractory status dystonicus in childhood. Dev Med Child Neurol 2014;56(7):649–56.

70. Elkay M, Silver K, Penn RD, et al. Dystonic storm due to Batten's disease treated with pallidotomy and deep brain stimulation. Mov Disord 2009;24(7): 1048–53.

71. Kyriagis M, Grattan-Smith P, Scheinberg A, et al. Status dystonicus and Hallervorden-Spatz disease: treatment with intrathecal baclofen and pallidotomy. J Paediatr Child Health 2004;40(5–6):322–5.

72. Blomstedt P, Taira T, Hariz M. Rescue pallidotomy for dystonia through implanted deep brain stimulation electrode. Surg Neurol Int 2016;7(Suppl 35): S815–7.

73. Takeda N, Horisawa S, Taira T, et al. Radiofrequency lesioning through deep brain stimulation electrodes in patients with generalized dystonia. World Neurosurg 2018;115:220–4.

74. Horisawa S, Kawamata T, Taira T. Unilateral pallidotomy for blepharospasm refractory to botulinum toxin injections. Eur J Neurol 2017;24(7):e39–40.

75. Horisawa S, Fukui A, Kohara K, et al. Unilateral pallidotomy in the treatment of cervical dystonia: a retrospective observational study. J Neurosurg 2021;134(1):216–21.

76. Horisawa S, Oka M, Kawamata T, et al. Bilateral pallidotomy for embouchure dystonia. Eur J Neurol 2018;25(9):e108–9.

77. Horisawa S, Oka M, Kohara K, et al. Staged bilateral pallidotomy for dystonic camptocormia: case report. J Neurosurg 2018;131(3):839–42.

78. Horisawa S, Fukui A, Takeda N, et al. Safety and efficacy of unilateral and bilateral pallidotomy for primary dystonia. Ann Clin Transl Neurol 2021;8(4): 857–65.

79. Centen LM, Oterdoom DLM, Tijssen MAJ, et al. Bilateral pallidotomy for dystonia: a systematic review. Mov Disord 2021;36(3):547–57.

80. Deuschl G, Antonini A, Costa J, et al. European academy of neurology/movement disorder Society-European section guideline on the treatment of Parkinson's disease: I. Invasive therapies. Mov Disord 2022;37(7):1360–74.

81. Hariz M, Bronstein JM, Cosgrove GR, et al. European Academy of Neurology/Movement Disorder Society-European Section Guidelines on Pallidotomy for Parkinson's Disease: Let's Be Accurate. Mov Disord 2022. https://doi.org/10.1002/mds. 29210. Online ahead of print.

82. 19th Biennial Meeting of the World Society for Stereotactic and Functional Neurosurgery, Incheon, Korea, September 4–7, 2022. Abstracts. In: Hodaie M, Chabardes S, Grenoble, et al, editors. Stereotact Funct Neurosurg 2022;100(suppl 1):3–370.

83. Ahmed AK, Guo S, Kelm N, et al. Technical comparison of treatment efficiency of magnetic resonance-guided focused ultrasound thalamotomy and pallidotomy in skull density ratio-matched patient cohorts. Front Neurol 2022;12:808810.

High-Frequency Ultrasound Ablation in Neurosurgery

Jonathan Pomeraniec, MD, MBA, W. Jeffrey Elias, MD*, Shayan Moosa, MD

KEYWORDS

- Focused ultrasound • High intensity • Magnetic resonance imaging • Thalamotomy

KEY POINTS

- High-intensity focused ultrasound techniques are increasingly used to create stereotactic ablations for medication-refractory movement and other neurologic disorders.
- Procedures have been shown to be safe and effective for essential tremor, Parkinson's disease, refractory pain, psychiatric disorders, and brain tumors.
- A growing number of stereotactic gray and white matter targets are being studied including ventrolateral and central lateral thalamus, pallidothalamic tract, globus pallidus, subthalamic nucleus, dentatorubrothalamic tract, and contralateral mesencephalon.
- Magnetic resonance-guided focused ultrasound procedures are generally well tolerated, and the most common adverse effects are largely mild and temporary.

INTRODUCTION

Although advances in imaging and lesioning technology have recently broadened the use of high-intensity focused ultrasound (HIFU) in neurosurgery,[1,2] the conceptualization of therapeutic uses for ultrasonography (US) in the central nervous system first occurred in the early 1950s. The kindred physicists William and Frank Fry illustrated the deep lesional effects of HIFU that left dura, intervening tissues, and blood vessels intact.[3,4] Eventual collaboration between the brothers and Russell Meyers, a pioneering surgeon of the basal ganglia, led to the study of thermal ablation for Parkinson's disease (PD) and other movement disorders.[5] Subsequent work led to the use of HIFU for glioma surgery after initial resection, as well as psychiatric and pain pathologies.[6] Despite early promise, the requirement of a craniotomy for acoustic transmission tempered adoption of US therapy in the neurosurgical community.

Modern transcranial magnetic resonance (MR)-guided focused ultrasound (MRgFUS) is an incisionless, ablative treatment modality for a growing number of neurologic disorders. This procedure selectively destroys a targeted volume of cerebral tissue and relies on real-time MR thermography to monitor tissue temperatures.[7,8] By focusing on a submillimeter target through a hemispheric phased array of transducers, ultrasound waves pass through the skull and avoid heating intervening structures.[1,9–11] Proprietary software used during the procedure minimizes phase distortion and aberrant ultrasound pathways that are byproducts of any skull irregularity.[12] Mechanical energy produced from ultrasound is subsequently absorbed by a volumetric target, converted into heat, and then causes focal destruction of brain tissue.[7]

PROCEDURE TECHNIQUE

Pre-operative volumetric computed tomography (CT) images are used to correct for ultrasound beam aberrations caused by inhomogeneity of the skull to ensure efficient delivery of individual

Department of Neurosurgery, University of Virginia, School of Medicine, PO Box 800212, Charlottesville, VA 22908, USA
* Corresponding author. Department of Neurological Surgery.
E-mail address: wje4r@uvahealth.org

1042-3680/23/© 2022 Elsevier Inc. All rights reserved.

neurosurgery.theclinics.com

ultrasound elements. These images are also used to identify sinuses, calcifications, membranes, and other "no-pass regions" that would otherwise alter direct delivery of ultrasound. In addition, the CT scan is used for calculating the ratio of cortical to cancellous bone of the skull (SDR), which is a predictor of the efficiency of ultrasound transmission and subsequent thermal rise.[13] At our institution, we generally do not treat patients with an SDR < 0.4.

After prepping the patient for the procedure, a complete head shave is performed to minimize the presence of microbubbles that could result in cavitation and scalp burns. Next, a stereotactic frame is placed under local anesthesia with an orientation that maximizes the surface area of the skull. The frame is used to secure the patient's head in place on the MRI table. On top of the frame, a silicone membrane acts as a conduit attachment to the ultrasound transducer, as well to cool the scalp with circulating water. After being secured by the frame to the transducer, the patient is placed into the isocenter of the MRI bore (**Fig. 1**A, B).

Following patient setup and initial transducer positioning, a series of reference localizing MR T1-or T2-weighted images are acquired and fused to a pre-procedure CT scan. In the case of ventral intermediate (VIM) nucleus thalamotomy for essential tremor (ET) or tremor-dominant Parkinson's disease (TDPD), the anterior commissure (AC), posterior commissure (PC), and midline form a constellation of anatomic landmarks for target planning. Such stereotactic planning can either be automated by software and indirect targeting from the AC-PC line or manually targeted to a directly visualized structure.[14] A common thalamic target for tremor corresponds to coordinates that are 1/4 of the AC-PC distance anterior to the PC and 14 mm lateral to midline (**Fig. 1**C). Targets can be adjusted more laterally or dorsally in the case of large ventricles and low SDR scores, respectively. In some cases, thalamic targets can be based on diffusion tensor imaging (DTI) connectivity or the dentatorubrothalamic tract (DRT).[15]

Before the treatment phase, movement detection algorithms based on a reference scan and fiducial markers are set up and registered. These tools help to automatically detect patient movement relative to the focus of the transducer. Final fine tuning of the transducer location can also be made at this point to match the planned target within millimeter precision.

After patient positioning and target planning, there are three phases of treatment sonication including aligning the focus, verifying the target, and creating the therapeutic ablation. Low energy sonications

elicit a moderate temperature rise at first, typically resulting in peak temperatures less than 45°C that do not cause permanent tissue damage. MR thermography is used to assess and potentially adjust the precise location of thermal rise relative to the planned target. Once the focus is properly aligned, the prescribed energy dose can be gradually increased through different combinations of power and/or duration. Thermal neuromodulation in the range of 50°C to 55°C seems to elicit initial neurologic effects, including partial tremor suppression or paresthesia.[16] The last treatment phase consists of increasing acoustic energy to produce peak voxel temperatures in the therapeutic ablation range of 55°C to 60°C (**Fig. 1**D–F). Patient assessment, including symptom response and the presence of any side effects, remains paramount in guiding the extent of lesioning. To expand the lesion within the VIM nucleus, the thermal ablation can be safely enlarged dorsally from the original target.[17]

PATIENT CONSIDERATIONS

In general, patient candidacy has focused on those with contraindications or disfavor for deep brain stimulation surgery (eg, advanced age, medical comorbidities precluding anesthesia, and/or intolerance of electrode implantation or device programming). Typical criteria for good candidates undergoing MRgFUS:

- Asymmetric symptoms (or symptom severity) favoring unilateral treatment
- Ability to undergo prolonged MR imaging (no claustrophobia or MR-incompatible devices) and participate in clinical assessments during the procedure
- Willingness to undergo a full head shave
- Preference for an incisionless procedure due to age and/or medical comorbidities
- Aversion to having and managing a permanent neuromodulation device

CLINICAL USES
Essential tremor

Several pilot investigations introduced the feasibility of transcranial MRgFUS for medication-refractory essential tremor.[16,18,19] Our initial experience showed significant and immediate symptomatic relief in 15 patients treated with unilateral Vim thalamotomy.[16] These benefits were still present after 1 year with 75% reduction of hand tremor, 85% reduction of overall disability, and 66% improvement of patient-reported quality of life (**Fig. 1**G, H). Later, Lipsman and colleagues showed an 81% reduction of Clinical Rating Scale for Tremor (CRST) scores in 3 patients at 3 months after

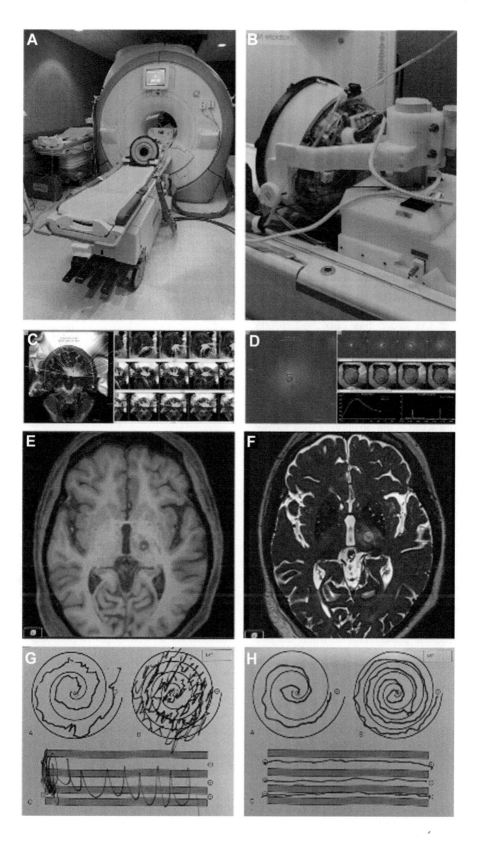

treatment.[19] Chang and colleagues verified these results although with mixed results of adequate thermal ablation in three of 11 patients.[18]

The Food and Drug Administration (FDA) approved unilateral MRgFUS thalamotomy for ET based on the results of a multicenter, randomized, double-blinded, sham-controlled clinical trial (**Table 1**). In this study, 56 patients were randomized to the treatment group, and 20 patients underwent a sham procedure. Patients in the treatment group experienced reduced tremor and disability scores by 47% and 59%, respectively, after 3 months, and these benefits remained sustained 1 year after the procedure.[20,21] The most common adverse events persisting 1 year following the procedure included gait disturbance in 14% of patients and paresthesias/numbness in 9%.[21,22] Long-term follow-up studies of patients from this cohort (who were not lost to follow-up at 2, 3, 4, and 5 years postoperatively) have shown sustained benefit.[18,23–25] Our group has published results from a survey of 85 patients with ET treated using MRgFUS thalamotomy with a mean follow-up of 3 years, demonstrating a 66% improvement in patient-reported tremor severity and 73% meaningful change in their overall condition. Of note, 89% of patients reported that they would repeat the procedure again in the position of their former selves.[10]

In addition to thalamic ablation, both Schreglmann and colleagues and Gallay and colleagues showed comparable promise of treating the more posteriorly located cerebellothalamic tract.[26,27] With diffusion-based tractography and stereotactic atlases, other groups have corroborated these findings and the utility of fiber imaging techniques.[9,28–30]

Parkinson's disease

Pallidothalamic tract

One of the earliest thermal ablations for 13 PD patients targeted the pallidothalamic tract. Magara and colleagues targeted the dense bundle of white matter fibers connecting the globus pallidus to the thalamus. As the pallidothalamic tract connects the pallidum to the thalamus and "densely packed axons, protected by their myelin sheaths, may indeed need a stronger thermal application than a loose nuclear target, composed of cell bodies, astrocytes, and extracellular matrix," the authors reported positive results only after increasing the energy thresholds in the latter half of the patient cohort.[31]

Ventrolateral thalamus

In 2017, our group continued work on Vim thalamotomy for tremor.[32] We found that patients suffering from refractory tremor (albeit ET, PD, or a smaller subset of patients with longstanding ET who later develop PD symptoms) can be safely and effectively treated by using the same target.[33–37] Three pilot studies of MRgFUS Vim thalamotomy showed that patients with PD experienced similar improvement of symptoms and overall quality of life.[32,36–38]

These findings were later confirmed by a multicenter, sham-controlled, randomized trial of 27 patients (20 randomized to MRgFUS thalamotomy and 7 to a sham procedure). Median tremor severity, as measured by the CRST Parts A + B, was significantly reduced in the "on" medication state for the treated cohort (62%) compared with the sham group (22%) after 3 months.[32] A recent study of patients with 1 to 5 years (median 36 months) of follow-up after thalamotomy showed significantly decreased CRST and UPDRS (Unified Parkinson's Disease Rating Scale) scores. Tremor returned completely in 7.7% of patients and partially in 30% of patients. Adverse effects were mild and transient.[39] MRgFUS thalamotomy was approved by the FDA for patients with tremor-dominant PD in 2018.

Reviewing single-center experience of thalamotomy for 160 consecutive procedures (of both

Figure 1. Transcranial magnetic resonance image-guided focused ultrasound (MRgFUS) thalamotomy. This is an example of MRgFUS for a left Vim thalamotomy in a 65-year-old female patient with tremor-dominant Parkinson's disease. (A) Commercial FUS system at our institution in a modified MR environment with a (B) magnified view of the silicone membrane affixed to an ultrasound transducer phased array consisting of 1024 elements that can focus high-intensity acoustic waves to an intracranial target. (C) Planning the target based on the AC-PC plane with 887 focused transducer elements. (D) MR thermography during the procedure showing thermal rise after a treatment sonication of 8400 J with a peak and average temperature curve to 65°C and 61°C, respectively. Red voxels indicate areas of temperature above a certain threshold. Post-procedure imaging on post-procedure day one showing the thermal ablation with surrounding edema in axial (E) T1-weighted and (F) T2-weighted magnetic resonance images. Archimedes spiral and line drawings (G) before and (H) after the procedure showing marked reduction in right hand tremor. AC, anterior commissure; MR, magnetic resonance; MRgFUS, magnetic resonance image-guided focused ultrasound; PC, posterior commissure; Vim, ventral intermediate nucleus of thalamus.

Table 1
Randomized controlled trials using transcranial magnetic resonance-guided focused ultrasound for the treatment of essential tremor and Parkinson's disease

First Author, Year	Number of Patients	Diagnosis	Target	Outcome at Primary Outcome Point	Persistent Adverse Effects at Last Follow-Up
Elias et al,[20] 2016	76 (56 treated, 20 sham)	ET	Vim	Hand CRST improved 47% at 3 mo	Paresthesias in 14% and imbalance in 9% at 12 mo
Bond et al,[32] 2017	27 (20 treated, 7 sham)	TDPD	Vim	Hand CRST improved 62% at 3 mo	Paresthesias in 20%, mild hemiparesis in 10%, and imbalance in 5% at 3 mo
Martinez-Fernandez et al,[47] 2020	40 (27 treated, 13 sham)	PD	STN	UPDRS III improved 50% at 4 mo	New-onset dyskinesia in 7%, mild hemiparesis in 7%, imbalance in 4%, and speech disturbance in 4% at 12 mo
Unpublished (NCT03319485)	91 (67 treated, 24 sham)	PD	GPi	UDysRS improved 47.5% and UPDRS III improved 26.4% at 3 mo	Dysarthria in 2.9%, facial drooping in 1.5%, gait imbalance in 1.5%, and numbness/paresthesias in 1.5%

Abbreviations: CRST, clinical rating scale for tremor; ET, essential tremor; GPi, globus pallidus internus; PD, Parkinson's disease; STN, subthalamic nucleus; TDPD, tremor-dominant Parkinson's disease; UDysRS, unified dyskinesia rating scale; UPDRS III, Unified Parkinson's Disease Rating Scale (part III); Vim, ventral intermediate nucleus.

ET and PD patients), Cosgrove and colleagues reported that all adverse effects were mild and diminished over time. The next day after the procedure, the most common adverse effects were imbalance (57%), sensory changes (25%) and dysmetria (11%). After 2 years, these effects improved to 18%, 10% and 8%, respectively.[40]

Globus pallidus pars interna

For patients with advanced motor fluctuations and medication-induced dyskinesia, the globus pallidus pars interna remains a common target for stereotactic modulation through deep brain stimulation and/or ablation. Na and colleagues first published results of unilateral focused ultrasound pallidotomy for PD. Symptoms were effectively suppressed for the first several series of patients, though there was later a report of dysarthria and contralateral hemiparesis after sonication likely owing to a lesional spread into the internal capsule.[41–44] Jung and colleagues performed a pilot study of 10 patients and found that all patients with follow-up at 6 months experienced significant improvement of UPDRS "off" medication scores.[44]

More recently, a pilot study of MRgFUS pallidotomy including 20 patients with PD has shown 59%

immediate improvement in the Unified Dyskinesia Rating Scale (UDysRS) with similar benefit 1 year following the procedure. Adverse events were all mild and transient.[45] A multi-center, sham-controlled, randomized trial to evaluate the safety and efficacy of unilateral pallidotomy for dyskinesia and/or motor fluctuations for advanced idiopathic PD (ClinicalTrials.gov Identifier: NCT03319485) has recently been completed, although the results are not yet published in a peer-reviewed journal. Among the 91 patients included in the study, 67 were treated with MRgFUS pallidotomy and 24 underwent a sham procedure. The treatment group showed a 68.6% response rate at 3 months following the procedure as compared with 33.3% in the sham group (a patient was considered a responder if they showed an improvement of more than three points in the off-medication UPDRS Part III or UDysRS scores without significant worsening of the other score). In the treatment group, UDysRS scores improved 47.5% and off-medication UPDRS part III scores improved by 26.4% 3 months after the procedure. Most adverse events were considered mild or moderate (91%), and the rates of dysarthria, facial drooping, gait imbalance, and numbness/tingling 12 months after the procedure were 2.9%, 1.5%, 1.5%, and 1.5%, respectively. Of note, MRgFUS pallidotomy was recently approved by the FDA for the treatment of motor symptoms associated with PD.

Subthalamic nucleus

Conceptually, the subthalamic nucleus would be an ideal target for MRI-guided HIFU ablation because it can be directly visualized as a small nucleus with potent antiparkinsonian effects. In 2018, a pilot study of 10 patients with advanced PD and asymmetric symptoms showed significant improvement of akinesia (88% reduction) and rigidity (23% reduction) up to 6 months after treatment. Side effects were minimal, with transient upper limb dyskinesia in two patients (one off-medication and one new onset, on-medication) at 6 months that resolved with titration of baseline medications.[46] In a multicenter, prospective, randomized, sham-controlled study of MRgFUS subthalamotomy for 40 patients with PD (27 treated and 13 sham), Martinez-Fernandez and colleagues showed a 10-point decrease in UPDRS III scores (from 19.9 to 9.9) 4 months after the procedure, with no significant change in the sham group.[46,47] New-onset speech disturbance, dyskinesia, weakness, and gait disturbance were observed in 11%, 11%, 7%, and 7% of patients 4 months after the procedure, respectively. This procedure is not currently approved by the FDA for the treatment of PD symptoms.

Pain

Chronic or persistent pain lasts longer than 12 weeks and often relapses and remits to wield longer-term disability.[48] To treat such long-lasting pain, thalamotomy, mesencephalotomy, and cingulotomy have achieved varied results.[49] For chronic neuropathic pain, a central lateral thalamotomy has been used to alleviate both somatosensory and affective elements of pain.[50] In a preliminary phase I study of 11 patients with chronic therapy-resistant neuropathic pain, mean pain relief was 49% and 57% at 3 months and 1 year follow-up periods, respectively. As a response to a symptomatic hemorrhage of the thalamus, additional safety measures were taken to include passive cavitation detection as well as auto-limited peak temperatures from sonication.[50]

Central lateral thalamotomy for trigeminal neuralgia has also been explored. In 2020, Gallay and colleagues showed safety and efficacy of disrupting the thalamocortical (TC) and corticocortical networks underlying the sensory, cognitive, and affective aspects of pain. The authors found 78% mean pain relief over 53 months.[51] Our group has completed a randomized, sham-controlled

trial of bilateral central lateral thalamotomy in 10 patients with chronic trigeminal neuropathic pain, which did not show the same degree of benefit observed in other studies (unpublished data).

Finally, there is a current investigation of the safety and efficacy of MRgFUS mesencephalotomy for refractory pain in patients with head and neck cancer (ClinicalTrials.gov Identifier: NCT03894553).

Psychiatric disease

Over the years, the underlying drive to root psychosurgery more empirically has ushered along the inspection of stereotactic ablation for major depressive disorder (MDD) and obsessive-compulsive disorder (OCD).[1,9] MR-guided bilateral thermal capsulotomy was tested as a proof-of-concept for treatment-refractory OCD in 2015 and then for MDD 3 years later.[52,53] To treat these refractory mental disorders, the authors targeted a region superior to the ventral striatum along the anterior limb of the internal capsule. The intention of this kind of ablation was to disrupt the putative network consisting of the striatum, thalamus, orbitofrontal, and cingulate cortex.[54,55] Throughout a 2-year follow-up period, a majority of 15 patients with OCD (split between two studies) experienced partial or full response without any durable adverse from ablation.[52] In 2018, Kim and colleagues showed a marked improvement of patient-reported depression scales in a 56-year-old woman with longstanding treatment-resistant MDD.[53]

More recently, Davidson and colleagues explored the clinical and imaging responses of bilateral anterior capsulotomy in patients with refractory OCD and MDD in two phase 1 trials. Half of the total patient cohort (4/6 OCD, 2/6 MDD) showed a positive response, and there were no reported serious adverse events over the course of follow-up. Using a combination of MRI-based structural connectome and positron emission tomography analysis, capsulotomy showed both targeted and widespread white-matter changes.[56,57]

Brain tumors

Less invasive treatment modalities of primary and metastatic brain tumors continue to expand.[58-64] Preliminary accounts of ultrasound ablation coupled with computed tomography guidance for malignant central nervous system tumors date back to the late 1980s.[6,65] About 20 years later, Ram and colleagues used HIFU with MR for three patients with recurrent high-grade glioma.[66,67] This initial experience came at a time of early transducer technology and was used to patients with craniotomy that permitted ultrasound waves to efficiently penetrate the brain. Soon thereafter in 2010,

McDannold and colleagues transmitted acoustic energy through intact skulls to treat high-grade gliomas of the thalamus.[68] These attempts resulted in modest intra-tumoral temperature rise, but fell short of thermal ablation in part due to technical limitations and a reduced number of transducer elements.[53] Four years later, Coluccia and colleagues reported the first safe and successful use of transcranial MRgFUS ablation, applying 25 high-power sonications in a 63-year-old patient with a centrally located recurrent glioblastoma.[69] Ongoing safety and feasibility trials of noninvasive thermal ablation for brain tumors are highlighting the inherent current limitations of MRgFUS, including relatively small and centrally located lesioning away from the skull (thereby precluding larger and peripheral tumor targets).[66,70]

COMPLICATIONS

Despite a few ingrained technical and biophysical limitations, MRgFUS continues to be an effective and well-tolerated procedure for patients with various neurologic disorders. The reported risk of serious side effects of this outpatient procedure is less than 2%.[22] For movement disorders, there are no reports of symptomatic intracerebral hemorrhage, infection, or mortality.[22] As mentioned earlier, the effects of cavitation and microbubble formation can be unpredictably untoward, but enhanced monitoring tools self-regulate these potential hazards. More common side effects include local head pain and face or limb paresthesias, which are typically transient. Less commonly, cerebellar symptoms like disequilibrium and/or ataxia can be elicited during the procedure, but these symptoms also largely resolve within weeks.[16] In terms of lasting positive effects, the overall treatment effect may decrease over time. This trajectory of results seems similar to other lesioning methods. Importantly, though, salvage therapy after failed or short-lasting focused ultrasound therapy can be done with DBS or repeat ablation.[71] As with any nascent treatment paradigm that grows with technological advance, HIFU procedures face unique challenges, chief among them parameter optimization in patients with unfavorable SDR, lengthening the endurance of lesioning, and treating advanced bilateral symptomatology. Other difficulties related to patient comfort include full head shaving and sometimes lengthy procedure times.[1,10,11,72]

FUTURE DIRECTIONS

The growing precision of pre-procedural planning and intra-procedural tools will likely warrant bilateral thalamotomies for tremor.[73] A current prospective, multi-site, single-arm, open-label study is evaluating the safety and efficacy of bilateral staged Exablate treatment in subjects with bilateral medication-refractory ET (ClinicalTrials. gov Identifier: NCT03465761).

Going forward, supplementary imaging modalities will help to improve the treatment and safety profile of HFIU procedures. Already, prospective MRI tractography for MRgFUS thalamotomy targeting affords enhanced visualization of white matter bundles coursing near the thalamus, including the medial lemniscus, corticospinal tract, and DRT.[29,30] Innovation in MR thermography and specialized multiple-echo spiral thermometry may open doors for real-time ablation monitoring in three dimensions.[74]

CLINICS CARE POINTS

- Thermal neuromodulation in the range of 50°C to 55°C wields initial neurologic effects, including partial tremor suppression or paresthesia. Higher energy doses that produce temperature curves in the range of 55°C to 60°C create therapeutic ablation.

- Magnetic resonance-guided focused ultrasound (MRgFUS) can be an appropriate treatment for patients with asymmetric symptoms (or symptom severity) favoring unilateral treatment, who are able to undergo prolonged MRI (no claustrophobia or MR-incompatible devices) and participate in clinical assessments during the procedure, and who are willing to undergo a full head shave.

- Intraprocedural MR thermography can be used to assess and potentially adjust the precise location of thermal rise relative to the planned target. Patient assessment, including symptom response and any durable side effects, remains paramount in guiding the extent of lesioning.

- For patients with essential tremor treated with MRgFUS thalamotomy, 3-year outcomes include 66% improvement in patient-reported tremor severity, 73% meaningful change in overall condition, and 89% of patients would repeat the original procedure

- The effects of cavitation and microbubble formation can be unpredictably untoward, but enhanced monitoring tools self-regulate these potential hazards. More common side effects include local head pain and face or limb paresthesias, which are typically transient. Less commonly, cerebellar symptoms like disequilibrium and/or ataxia can be elicited during the procedure, but these symptoms also largely resolve within weeks.

DISCLOSURE

Dr Elias serves as a consultant for Insightec, Ltd. The other authors have nothing to disclose. There are no funding sources associated with this manuscript.

REFERENCES

1. Franzini A, Moosa S, Servello D, et al. Ablative brain surgery: an overview. Int J Hyperthermia 2019;36(2): 64–80.
2. Elias WJ, Khaled M, Hilliard JD, et al. A magnetic resonance imaging, histological, and dose modeling comparison of focused ultrasound, radiofrequency, and Gamma Knife radiosurgery lesions in swine thalamus. J Neurosurg 2013;119(2):307–17.
3. Fry WJ, Barnard JW, Fry EJ, et al. Ultrasonic lesions in the mammalian central nervous system. Science 1955;122(3168):517–8.
4. Fry WJ, Mosberg WH Jr, Barnard JW, et al. Production of focal destructive lesions in the central nervous system with ultrasound. J Neurosurg 1954; 11(5):471–8.
5. Fry FJ, Ades HW, Fry WJ. Production of reversible changes in the central nervous system by ultrasound. Science 1958;127(3289):83–4.
6. Heimburger RF. Ultrasound augmentation of central nervous system tumor therapy. Indiana Med 1985; 78(6):469–76.
7. Haar GT, Coussios C. High intensity focused ultrasound: physical principles and devices. Int J Hyperthermia 2007;23(2):89–104.
8. Gazelle GS, Goldberg SN, Solbiati L, et al. Tumor ablation with radio-frequency energy. Radiology 2000;217(3):633–46.
9. Franzini A, Moosa S, Prada F, et al. Ultrasound ablation in neurosurgery: current clinical applications and future perspectives. Neurosurgery 2020;87(1): 1–10.
10. Moosa S, Craver A, Asuzu D, et al. Patient-reported outcomes and predictive factors following focused ultrasound thalamotomy for essential tremor. Stereotact Funct Neurosurg 2022;1–9. https://doi.org/10.1159/000525763.
11. Moosa S, Martinez-Fernandez R, Elias WJ, et al. The role of high-intensity focused ultrasound as a symptomatic treatment for Parkinson's disease. Mov Disord 2019;34(9):1243–51.
12. Colen RR, Sahnoune I, Weinberg JS. Neurosurgical Applications of High-Intensity Focused Ultrasound

with Magnetic Resonance Thermometry. Neurosurg Clin N Am 2017;28(4):559–67.
13. Boutet A, Gwun D, Gramer R, et al. The relevance of skull density ratio in selecting candidates for transcranial MR-guided focused ultrasound. J Neurosurg 2019;132(6):1785–91.
14. Schaltenbrand G, Bailey P. Einfuhrung in die stereotaktischen Operationen, mit einem Atlas des menschlichen Gehirns. Introduction to stereotaxis, with an atlas of the human brain. Stuttgart: Thieme; 1959.
15. Sammartino F, Krishna V, King NK, et al. Tractography-Based Ventral Intermediate Nucleus Targeting: Novel Methodology and Intraoperative Validation. Mov Disord 2016;31(8):1217–25.
16. Elias WJ, Huss D, Voss T, et al. A pilot study of focused ultrasound thalamotomy for essential tremor. N Engl J Med 2013;369(7):640–8.
17. Wang TR, Bond AE, Dallapiazza RF, et al. Transcranial magnetic resonance imaging-guided focused ultrasound thalamotomy for tremor: technical note. Neurosurg Focus 2018;44(2):E3.
18. Chang WS, Jung HH, Kweon EJ, et al. Unilateral magnetic resonance guided focused ultrasound thalamotomy for essential tremor: practices and clinicoradiological outcomes. J Neurol Neurosurg Psychiatry 2015;86(3):257–64.
19. Lipsman N, Schwartz ML, Huang Y, et al. MR-guided focused ultrasound thalamotomy for essential tremor: a proof-of-concept study. Lancet Neurol 2013;12(5):462–8.
20. Elias WJ. A trial of focused ultrasound thalamotomy for essential tremor. N Engl J Med 2016;375(22): 2202–3.
21. Elias WJ, Lipsman N, Ondo WG, et al. A randomized trial of focused ultrasound thalamotomy for essential tremor. N Engl J Med 2016;375(8):730–9.
22. Fishman PS, Elias WJ, Ghanouni P, et al. Neurological adverse event profile of magnetic resonance imaging-guided focused ultrasound thalamotomy for essential tremor. Mov Disord 2018;33(5):843–7.
23. Park YS, Jung NY, Na YC, et al. Four-year follow-up results of magnetic resonance-guided focused ultrasound thalamotomy for essential tremor. Mov Disord 2019;34(5):727–34.
24. Cosgrove GR, Lipsman N, Lozano AM, et al. Magnetic resonance imaging-guided focused ultrasound thalamotomy for essential tremor: 5-year follow-up results. J Neurosurg 2022;5:1–6.
25. Halpern CH, Santini V, Lipsman N, et al. Three-year follow-up of prospective trial of focused ultrasound thalamotomy for essential tremor. Neurology 2019; 93(24):e2284–93.
26. Gallay MN, Moser D, Rossi F, et al. Incisionless transcranial MR-guided focused ultrasound in essential tremor: cerebellothalamic tractotomy. J Ther Ultrasound 2016;4:5.

27. Schreglmann SR, Bauer R, Hagele-Link S, et al. Unilateral cerebellothalamic tract ablation in essential tremor by MRI-guided focused ultrasound. Neurology 2017;88(14):1329–33.

28. Chazen JL, Sarva H, Stieg PE, et al. Clinical improvement associated with targeted interruption of the cerebellothalamic tract following MR-guided focused ultrasound for essential tremor. J Neurosurg 2018;129(2):315–23.

29. Krishna V, Sammartino F, Agrawal P, et al. Prospective tractography-based targeting for improved safety of focused ultrasound thalamotomy. Neurosurgery 2019;84(1):160–8.

30. Tian Q, Wintermark M, Jeffrey Elias W, et al. Diffusion MRI tractography for improved transcranial MRI-guided focused ultrasound thalamotomy targeting for essential tremor. Neuroimage Clin 2018;19: 572–80.

31. Magara A, Buhler R, Moser D, et al. First experience with MR-guided focused ultrasound in the treatment of Parkinson's disease. J Ther Ultrasound 2014;2:11.

32. Bond AE, Shah BB, Huss DS, et al. Safety and efficacy of focused ultrasound thalamotomy for patients with medication-refractory, tremor-dominant parkinson disease: a randomized clinical trial. JAMA Neurol 2017;74(12):1412–8.

33. Dallapiazza RF, Lee DJ, De Vloo P, et al. Outcomes from stereotactic surgery for essential tremor. J Neurol Neurosurg Psychiatry 2019;90(4):474–82.

34. Fasano A, De Vloo P, Llinas M, et al. Magnetic resonance imaging-guided focused ultrasound thalamotomy in parkinson tremor: reoperation after benefit decay. Mov Disord 2018;33(5):848–9.

35. Ito H, Fukutake S, Yamamoto K, et al. Magnetic resonance imaging-guided focused ultrasound thalamotomy for parkinson's disease. Intern Med 2018; 57(7):1027–31.

36. Schlesinger I, Eran A, Sinai A, et al. MRI guided focused ultrasound thalamotomy for moderate-to-severe tremor in parkinson's disease. Parkinsons Dis 2015;2015:219149.

37. Zaaroor M, Sinai A, Goldsher D, et al. Magnetic resonance-guided focused ultrasound thalamotomy for tremor: a report of 30 Parkinson's disease and essential tremor cases. J Neurosurg 2018;128(1): 202–10.

38. Fasano A, Llinas M, Munhoz RP, et al. MRI-guided focused ultrasound thalamotomy in non-ET tremor syndromes. Neurology 2017;89(8):771–5.

39. Sinai A, Nassar M, Sprecher E, et al. Focused ultrasound thalamotomy in tremor dominant parkinson's disease: long-term results. J Parkinsons Dis 2022; 12(1):199–206.

40. Lak AM, Segar DJ, McDannold N, et al. Magnetic resonance image guided focused ultrasound thalamotomy. a single center experience with 160 procedures. Front Neurol 2022;13:743649.

41. Alkhani A, Lozano AM. Pallidotomy for parkinson disease: a review of contemporary literature. J Neurosurg 2001;94(1):43–9.

42. de Bie RM, de Haan RJ, Nijssen PC, et al. Unilateral pallidotomy in Parkinson's disease: a randomised, single-blind, multicentre trial. Lancet 1999;354(9191): 1665–9.

43. Na YC, Chang WS, Jung HH, et al. Unilateral magnetic resonance-guided focused ultrasound pallidotomy for Parkinson disease. Neurology 2015; 85(6):549–51.

44. Jung NY, Park CK, Kim M, et al. The efficacy and limits of magnetic resonance-guided focused ultrasound pallidotomy for Parkinson's disease: a Phase I clinical trial. J Neurosurg 2018;1–9. https://doi.org/ 10.3171/2018.2.JNS172514.

45. Eisenberg HM, Krishna V, Elias WJ, et al. MR-guided focused ultrasound pallidotomy for Parkinson's disease: safety and feasibility. J Neurosurg 2020;27: 1–7.

46. Martinez-Fernandez R, Rodriguez-Rojas R, Del Alamo M, et al. Focused ultrasound subthalamotomy in patients with asymmetric Parkinson's disease: a pilot study. Lancet Neurol 2018;17(1): 54–63.

47. Martinez-Fernandez R, Manez-Miro JU, Rodriguez-Rojas R, et al. Randomized trial of focused ultrasound subthalamotomy for parkinson's disease. N Engl J Med 2020;383(26):2501–13.

48. Treede RD, Rief W, Barke A, et al. A classification of chronic pain for ICD-11. Pain 2015;156(6):1003–7.

49. Menon JP. Intracranial ablative procedures for the treatment of chronic pain. Neurosurg Clin N Am 2014;25(4):663–70.

50. Jeanmonod D, Werner B, Morel A, et al. Transcranial magnetic resonance imaging-guided focused ultrasound: noninvasive central lateral thalamotomy for chronic neuropathic pain. Neurosurg Focus 2012; 32(1):E1.

51. Gallay MN, Moser D, Jeanmonod D. MR-guided focused ultrasound central lateral thalamotomy for trigeminal neuralgia. single center experience. Front Neurol 2020;11:271.

52. Jung HH, Kim SJ, Roh D, et al. Bilateral thermal capsulotomy with MR-guided focused ultrasound for patients with treatment-refractory obsessive-compulsive disorder: a proof-of-concept study. Mol Psychiatry 2015;20(10):1205–11.

53. Kim M, Kim CH, Jung HH, et al. Treatment of major depressive disorder via magnetic resonance-guided focused ultrasound surgery. Biol Psychiatry 2018;83(1):e17–8.

54. Brown LT, Mikell CB, Youngerman BE, et al. Dorsal anterior cingulotomy and anterior capsulotomy for severe, refractory obsessive-compulsive disorder: a systematic review of observational studies. J Neurosurg 2016;124(1):77–89.

55. Patel SR, Aronson JP, Sheth SA, et al. Lesion procedures in psychiatric neurosurgery. World Neurosurg 2013;80(3–4):S31 e9–31 e16.

56. Davidson B, Hamani C, Meng Y, et al. Examining cognitive change in magnetic resonance-guided focused ultrasound capsulotomy for psychiatric illness. Transl Psychiatry 2020;10(1):397.

57. Davidson B, Hamani C, Rabin JS, et al. Magnetic resonance-guided focused ultrasound capsulotomy for refractory obsessive compulsive disorder and major depressive disorder: clinical and imaging results from two phase I trials. Mol Psychiatry 2020; 25(9):1946–57.

58. Anzai Y, Lufkin R, DeSalles A, et al. Preliminary experience with MR-guided thermal ablation of brain tumors. AJNR Am J Neuroradiol 1995;16(1):39–48 [discussion: 49-52].

59. Ashraf O, Patel NV, Hanft S, et al. Laser-induced thermal therapy in neuro-oncology: a review. World Neurosurg 2018;112:166–77.

60. Kondziolka D, Flickinger JC, Lunsford LD. Stereotactic radiosurgery for epilepsy and functional disorders. Neurosurg Clin N Am 2013;24(4):623–32.

61. Maroon JC, Onik G, Quigley MR, et al. Cryosurgery re-visited for the removal and destruction of brain, spinal and orbital tumours. Neurol Res 1992;14(4): 294–302.

62. Regis J. Gamma knife for functional diseases. Neurotherapeutics 2014;11(3):583–92.

63. Winter A, Laing J, Paglione R, et al. Microwave hyperthermia for brain tumors. Neurosurgery 1985; 17(3):387–99.

64. Yang I, Udawatta M, Prashant GN, et al. Stereotactic radiosurgery for neurosurgical patients: a historical review and current perspectives. World Neurosurg 2019;122:522–31.

65. Guthkelch AN, Carter LP, Cassady JR, et al. Treatment of malignant brain tumors with focused ultrasound hyperthermia and radiation: results of a phase I trial. J Neurooncol 1991;10(3):271–84.

66. Prada F, Kalani MYS, Yagmurlu K, et al. Applications of focused ultrasound in cerebrovascular diseases and brain tumors. Neurotherapeutics 2019;16(1): 67–87.

67. Ram Z, Cohen ZR, Harnof S, et al. Magnetic resonance imaging-guided, high-intensity focused ultrasound for brain tumor therapy. Neurosurgery 2006; 59(5):949–55 [discussion: 955-6].

68. McDannold N, Clement GT, Black P, et al. Transcranial magnetic resonance imaging- guided focused ultrasound surgery of brain tumors: initial findings in 3 patients. Neurosurgery 2010;66(2):323–32 [discussion: 332].

69. Coluccia D, Fandino J, Schwyzer L, et al. First noninvasive thermal ablation of a brain tumor with MR-guided focused ultrasound. J Ther Ultrasound 2014;2:17.

70. Prada F, Vitale V, Del Bene M, et al. Contrast-enhanced MR Imaging versus Contrast-enhanced US: A Comparison in Glioblastoma Surgery by Using Intraoperative Fusion Imaging. Radiology 2017; 285(1):242–9.

71. Wang TR, Dallapiazza RF, Moosa S, et al. Thalamic deep brain stimulation salvages failed focused ultrasound thalamotomy for essential tremor: a case report. Stereotact Funct Neurosurg 2018;96(1):60–4.

72. Franzini A, Attuati L, Zaed I, et al. Gamma Knife central lateral thalamotomy for the treatment of neuropathic pain. J Neurosurg 2020;1–9. https://doi.org/ 10.3171/2020.4.JNS20558.

73. Alshaikh J, Fishman PS. Revisiting bilateral thalamotomy for tremor. Clin Neurol Neurosurg 2017; 158:103–7.

74. Marx M, Ghanouni P, Butts Pauly K. Specialized volumetric thermometry for improved guidance of MRgFUS in brain. Magn Reson Med 2017;78(2): 508–17.

Moving?

Make sure your subscription moves with you!

To notify us of your new address, find your **Clinics Account Number** (located on your mailing label above your name), and contact customer service at:

Email: journalscustomerservice-usa@elsevier.com

800-654-2452 (subscribers in the U.S. & Canada)
314-447-8871 (subscribers outside of the U.S. & Canada)

Fax number: 314-447-8029

Elsevier Health Sciences Division
Subscription Customer Service
3251 Riverport Lane
Maryland Heights, MO 63043

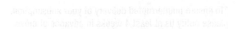

Printed and bound by CPI Group (UK) Ltd, Croydon, CR0 4YY

08/05/2025

01864750-0013